Effective Documentation for Physical Therapy Professionals

Notice

Medicine is an ever-changing science. As new research and clinical experience broaden our knowledge, changes in treatment and drug therapy are required. The authors and the publisher of this work have checked with sources believed to be reliable in their efforts to provide information that is complete and generally in accord with the standards accepted at the time of publication. However, in view of the possibility of human error or changes in medical sciences, neither the authors nor the publishers nor any other party who has been involved in the preparation or publication of this work warrants that the information contained herein is in every respect accurate or complete, and they disclaim all responsibility for any errors or omissions or for the results obtained from use of information contained in this work. Readers are encouraged to confirm the information contained herein with other sources. For example and in particular, readers are advised to check the product information sheet included in the package of each drug they plan to administer to be certain that the information contained in this work is accurate and that changes have not been made in the recommended dose or in the contraindications for administration. This recommendation is of particular importance in connection with the new or infrequently used drugs.

Effective Documentation for Physical Therapy Professionals

Eric Shamus, PT, PhD, CSCS
Assistant Professor
Osteopathic Principles and Practice
College of Osteopathic Medicine
Health Professions Division
Nova Southeastern University
Ft. Lauderdale, Florida

Debra Feingold Stern, PT, MSM, DBA
Assistant Professor of Physical Therapy
College of Allied Health
Health Professions Division
Nova Southeastern University
Ft. Lauderdale, Florida

McGraw-Hill
Medical Publishing Division

New York   Chicago   San Francisco   Lisbon   London   Madrid   Mexico City
Milan   New Delhi   San Juan   Seoul   Singapore   Sydney   Toronto

The McGraw·Hill Companies

Effective Documentation for Physical Therapy Professionals

Copyright © 2004 by the **McGraw-Hill Companies,** Inc. All rights reserved. Printed in the United States of America. Except as permitted under the United States Copyright Act of 1976, no part of this publication may be reproduced or distributed in any form or by any means, or stored in a database or retrieval system, without the prior written permission of the publisher.

234567890 VFMVFM 0987654

ISBN 0-07-140065-6

This book was set in Times Roman by Circle Graphics.
The editors were Michael Brown, Janene Matragrano, and Regina Y. Brown.
The production supervisor was Catherine H. Saggese.
The cover designer was Janice Bielawa.
The text designer was Marsha Cohen/Parallelogram Graphics.
The index was prepared by Robert Swanson.
Von Hoffmann was the printer and binder.

This book is printed on acid-free paper.

Cataloging-in-Publication Data is on file for this title at the Library of Congress.

Current Procedural Terminology (CPT) is copyright 2003 American
Medical Association. All Rights Reserved. No fee schedules, basic
units, relative values, or relating listings are included in CPT. The
AMA assumes no liability for the data contained herein. Applicable
FARS/DFARS restrictions apply to government use.

CPT® is a trademark of the American Medical Association.

**Please tell the author and publisher what you think of this book by sending your comments to pt@mcgraw-hill.com.
Please put the author and title of the book in the subject line.**

This book is dedicated to our families,

Allan, Margot, and Darren

and

Jennifer and Grant

For their love, support and guidance.

Contents

Contributors		*ix*
Preface		*xi*
Acknowledgments		*xiii*
Chapter 1	Introduction, Purpose, and General Rules for Health Information Management (Medical Record Keeping)	1
Chapter 2	Record Organization and General Principles	11
Chapter 3	Application of Models for Organization and Guidelines for Content	21
Chapter 4	Component Requirements	33
Chapter 5	Coding and Documentation	43
Chapter 6	Standardized Forms and Content	57
Chapter 7	Legal Issues in the Medical Record	71
Chapter 8	MDS Purpose and Components	91
Chapter 9	Medicare and Non-Medicare Content Principles	103
Chapter 10	Pediatric Documentation	123
Chapter 11	The Electronic Medical Record or Computerized Patient Record	139
Chapter 12	Utilization Review and Utilization Management	153
Pediatric References		177
Appendix A	Abbreviations	181
Appendix B	CMS 700 Form	197
Appendix C	CMS Forms 1450 and 1500 with Instructions	201
Appendix D	ICD-9 Code Terms	207
Appendix E	APTA Guidelines for Physical Therapy Documentation	211
Appendix F	Goal Writing Exercise	229
Appendix G	Note Writing Exercise	233
Appendix H	Documentation Content Exercise	237
Appendix I	Physical Therapy Note Examples	241
Index		253

Contributors

Keith E. Christianssen, PT, ATC, MTC
Director of Content Development for TherapySource
Owner of Competitive Edge Seminars
Birmingham, Alabama

Barbara Deering, PT
Director of URQA
Outreach Programs, Inc.
Ft. Lauderdale, Florida

Gerard G. Fluet, MSPT
Senior Physical Therapist
JFK-Johnson Rehabilitation Institute
Adjunct Professor
Department of Pediatrics and Rehabilitation
University of Medicine and Dentistry of New Jersey
Edison, New Jersey

Rebecca S. Rosenthal, PT, MS, JD
Assistant Professor of Physical Therapy
Physical Therapy Department
College of Allied Health
Health Professions Division
Nova Southeastern University
Ft. Lauderdale, Florida

Claudia Senesac, PT, PCS, MHS
Department of Physical Therapy
University of Florida
Gainesville, Florida

Kay H. Tasso, PT, PCS, MA, PhD
Assistant Professor of Physical Therapy
University of North Florida
Jacksonville, Florida

Preface

In a changing health care environment, Physical Therapists cannot afford third party payer denial for services they provide. Common reasons for denials include:

- **Technical errors such as:**
  - identifier omission
  - incorrect form use
  - incorrect information
  - inadequate information
- **Non-technical errors such as:**
  - illegibility
  - good documentation in wrong place
  - bad documentation anyplace
  - billing information does not match documentation of care
  - goals do not match problems or diagnosis
  - outcomes or effectiveness of therapy services for patient's illness or injury (i.e. goals not achieved) are not documented
  - patient achieved their restorative potential and were provided repetitive, non-skilled exercises
  - patient did not require the care of a skilled therapist based on documentation
  - loss of function or functional limitation was not identified (problems were physiologically impairment based)
  - potential for significant improvement not identified (goals were not significant enough to justify care, or patient was too high level or too low level)
  - need for skilled therapist not identified (improvement would have been made without therapeutic intervention)
  - maintenance type therapies being provided (rote, repetitive treatment to maintain same level of function)

Incorporating all of the general principles for documentation and health information management should help the therapist maintain records appropriately, organize the record, record appropriate information and receive reimbursement based on the documentation content. The therapist should seek to write only what is relevant and necessary and in an objective manner, using verbiage that indicates skill, but is universally understood based on all purposes of the medical record. By appreciating why payment for physical therapy services is denied, the therapist can reflect on documentation content guidelines and the importance of content adherence.

This textbook will help lay the foundation on What, How and Why to document. Legal Issues, Coding, Utilization Review and utilization management are just a few of the contents areas covered.

Acknowledgments

We would like to thank and acknowledge all the individuals who contributed to this book. Without their expertise and dedication, this book would not have been possible.

Special thanks to Julie Scardiglia and the McGraw Hill staff for their never ending help and encouragement.

Additional thanks to Dr. Cheryl Hill, Director of the Physical Therapy Department at Nova Southeastern University and Dean Rick Davis for their support, as well as Dr. Elaine Wallace, Dr. Michael Patterson and Dean Tony Silvagni of the College of Osteopathic Medicine. Special thanks to Frederick Lippman, B.Sc., R.Ph., Executive Vice Chancellor and Provost of the Health Professions Division of Nova Southeastern University.

Eric Shamus
Debra Feingold Stern

1

Introduction, Purpose, and General Rules for Health Information Management (Medical Record Keeping)

Introduction and Purposes of the Record

Physical therapy, although not known by name until modern times, has had a long history. Oral history, recorded information, documents, and archaeological discoveries enable us to trace the history of medical practice, including physical medicine practices through the ages. While some record keeping was important to previous generations, it is more so today, although modern standards did not appear until the twentieth century. The Hospital Standardization Program established the first requirement for "complete and accurate reporting of the care and treatment provided during hospitalization" in 1918.[1] Before 1918, individual physicians haphazardly maintained records according to their personal purpose and convenience, unless they were associated with research.

In some respects, the purposes for record keeping or documenting have remained constant. However, as the complexity of healthcare has grown, so has the management of medical information. Health Information Management (HIM) is replacing the term medical record keeping. The American Health Information Management Association is setting the standards for the overall science of HIM in an increasingly complex system. The patient chart/record itself is considered a legal document and is, therefore, subject to state and federal laws, as well as medical record laws and state licensure laws and acts.

For physical therapy professionals, as with other health professionals, documentation is a required practice by federal, state, facility, and accreditation laws and guidelines. Although required in all settings with some differing requirements, effective and efficient appropriate documentation that complies with all purposes and regulations can be vexing to the practitioner. Fundamentals are traditionally taught in the academic setting, but the principles learned during one's education need to be practically adapted and applied in the working world. Since style and required content vary among facilities, agencies, and therapists, practical application is more challenging than theoretical application.

When the Medicare program was established in 1966 with Title XVIII of the Social Security Act, physical therapy became a billable service. Under the Act, all practitioners are required to document patient care and often prove the medical necessity of care. At the time, most physical therapy was hospital-based for both in-patient and outpatient, and payment did not depend on record content. Regulations existed for documentation in the Medicare program for all outpatient and skilled inpatient rehabilitation services as early as the 1970s (and remain in effect today). From a technical perspective, all delivered services required physician prescription or referral, ongoing physician visits, and justification of care as evidenced by documentation. Depending on the setting, hospital, skilled nursing, outpatient, or home health, reimbursement was on a fee-for-service or cost-based basis. In fee-for-service arrangements, rare in the twenty-first century, providers charged a fee and the third-party payer paid, assuming the fees were reasonable and customary in the community. Cost-based reimbursement was derived from the costs incurred by the organization without regard for preset parameters, but rather categories that were acceptable for reimbursement: skilled nursing facilities, rehabilitation agencies, certified outpatient rehabilitation (CARF).

The 1970s was also a time of increasing medical malpractice claims. Since the only evidence of care after patient discharge was the written medical record, the record content became crucial in proving innocence (or potential guilt) of the healthcare provider. Although the number of malpractice suits against physical therapists was and continues to be small, it continues to be the documentation that supports innocence and protects or potentially contributes to convicting the provider.

Before healthcare costs began escalating in the 1970s and 1980s, documentation content was not used to any extent to deny reimbursement to the provider, as neither the federal government nor private industry had the technology to properly track claims. However, in the 1980s, with the advent of computerization, Medicare was able to track services for the first time. As this became possible, the Healthcare Finance Administration (HCFA, now Center for Medicare and Medicaid, CMS), embarked on a program to uncover fraud and abuse for all Medicare-provided services, including physical therapy (PT). In the early 1990s, commercial payers determined that they could also track services and determine if documentation supported the care rendered. Tracking resulted in recovery of millions of dollars from fraudulent claims in the 1980s and 1990s, and continues today.

The healthcare delivery system has evolved into a managed care–oriented system in the early twenty-first century. As the healthcare industry continues to experience incremental reform, managed care—the initiative that seeks to deliver appropriate and cost-effective healthcare without sacrificing quality—demands an effective and efficient billing tracking process. Decreases in reimbursement by third-party payers within a managed care environment, whether by decreased dollars per visit, visit limitation, or capitation, have forced physical therapists to ensure reimbursement of all available funds through documentation. The documentation must justify care that reflects the need for skilled services, be concise and accurate (effective and efficient), and match all billing information with correct coding. According to Stewart and Abeln, 1993, "Carriers do not place a high value on physical therapy services as they relate to managed care concepts."[2] Therefore, the burden falls to the physical therapist (PT) to justify the value.

Medicare, administered by the Centers for Medicare and Medicaid (CMS), formerly Healthcare Financing Administration (HCFA), a division of Health and Human Services (HHS), one of the largest payers in healthcare, dictates basic content for documentation for rehabilitation professionals, including physical therapists. Data gathered by CMS are maintained in a national database where it is stored and analyzed and used to "make decisions related to healthcare reimbursement mechanisms, the effectiveness of healthcare services, and the general health of the Medicare population."[3] The state government (Medicaid) and other third-party payers maintain similar data for decision-making purposes. However, since a fiscal intermediary (FI) contracted with CMS administers payment to the care provider, the regulations are open to interpretation by the payer as well as the care provider. The one constant is that services must be skilled in nature and justified.

Physical therapists (PTs) have historically been lax in making the connection in their documentation between the medical problem, the PT-related functional problem or PT diagnosis, the PT treatment, and objective measures of outcomes. PTs have been challenged in relating treatment and goals to function, and providing evidence that PT is better than alternative patient management. Documentation content has been primarily impairment based, focusing on the physiology of a problem. As a result, PT has not been considered an essential medical service. With the current movement within the profession for evidenced-based practice, the future may be different. The APTA's *Guide to Physical Therapist Practice* stresses these relationships.

Consistent terminology both in description and content is also a challenge for the physical therapist. The American Health Information Management Association (AHIMA) uses the general term health record to categorize what may be more commonly known, depending on setting, as the patient records (acute care), medical records (physician offices, physical therapy practices/departments), resident records (skilled nursing facilities), or client records (ambulatory care, American Physical Therapy Association). A health record contains all information about the patient/client including the skilled documentation. The *Guide to Physical Therapist Practice,* 2nd edition refers to documentation as a role of the physical therapist. Documentation is defined in the Guide as "any entry into the client record, such as consultation report, initial examination report, progress note, flow sheet/checklist that identifies the care/service provided, reexamination, or summation of care."[4] Colloquially, physical therapists are familiar with the term medical record, because the Guide terminology was only recently developed. Regardless of the terminology, the record is "the principal repository (storage place) for data and information about the healthcare services provided to an individual patient. It documents the who, what, when, where, what, and how of patient care."[5]

It is interesting and important to note that historically, documentation has been by manual entry with maintenance of a hard copy record. To increase speed and efficiency, dictation and transcription were introduced in the twentieth century. Though costly and more commonly used by physicians, the practice of dictation and transcription was also adopted by physical therapists (primarily in the outpatient setting) for the same purpose. As we enter the twenty-first century, the future of recording and record keeping continues to evolve. The computer-based patient record (CPR) or electronic medical record (EMR) is gaining popularity. Whether an entry is made simply with a word processing program or through a custom-designed integrated record system, hard copy or paper records may soon become part of history. However, regardless of whether a professional uses a pen or keyboard, narrative, SOAP format (subjective, objective, assessment, plan), or templates, the general principles, purposes, and content requirements remain the same.

Functions and Users of the Health Record

According to AHIMA, the basic purposes of documentation are: (1) to serve as a basis for planning and treatment; (2) a means of communication for attending health professionals; (3) as legal entries describing the care the patient receives; (4) verification of services for payers, and (5) as basic data for health research and planning. The Institute of Medicine[6] divides the purposes into primary and secondary, where primary purposes directly relate to patient care (See Table 1.1) and secondary purposes indirectly relate to patient care (See Table 1.2).

The primary purposes identified by the Institute are patient care delivery, patient care management, patient care support, and billing and reimbursement. *Patient care delivery* is the care provided by the professionals involved in a patient's care. This is used by the providers to communicate what is being done and the outcome or patient response to treatment in order to ensure continuity of care. To this end, it is imperative

Table 1.1
PRIMARY PURPOSES
OF THE HEALTH
RECORD

Patient Care Delivery (Patient)

- To document services received
- To constitute proof of identity
- To self-manage care
- To verify billing

Patient Care Delivery (Provider)

- To foster continuity of care (that is, to serve as a communication tool)
- To describe diseases and causes (that is, to support diagnostic work)
- To support decision making about diagnosis and treatment of patients
- To assess and manage risk for individual patients
- To facilitate care in accordance with clinical practice guidelines
- To document patient risk factors
- To assess and document patient expectations and patient satisfaction
- To generate care plans
- To determine preventive advice or health maintenance information
- To provide reminders to clinicians
- To support nursing care
- To document services provided

Patient Care Management

- To document case mix in institutions and practices
- To analyze severity of illness
- To formulate practice guidelines
- To manage risk
- To characterize the use of services
- To provide the basis for utilization review
- To perform quality assurance

Patient Care Support

- To allocate resources
- To analyze trends and develop forecasts
- To assess workload
- To communicate information among departments

Billing and Reimbursement

- To document services for payments
- To bill for services
- To submit insurance claims
- To adjudicate insurance claims
- To determine disabilities (for example, workman's compensation)
- To manage costs
- To report costs
- To perform actuarial analysis

SOURCE: Dick, Steen, and Detmer 1997, p. 78.

Table 1.2
SECONDARY
PURPOSES OF
THE HEALTH
RECORD

Education

- To document the experience of healthcare professionals
- To prepare conferences and presentations
- To teach healthcare students

Regulation

- To serve as evidence in litigation
- To foster postmarketing surveillance
- To assess compliance with standards of care
- To accredit professionals and hospitals
- To compare healthcare organizations

Research

- To develop new products
- To conduct clinical research
- To assess technology
- To study patient outcomes
- To study effectiveness and cost-effectiveness of patient care
- To identify populations at risk
- To develop registries and databases
- To assess the cost-effectiveness of record systems

Policy Making

- To allocate resources
- To conduct strategic planning
- To monitor public health

Industry

- To conduct research and development
- To plan marketing strategy

SOURCE: Dick, Steen, and Detmer 1997, p. 79.

that the record be available as needed to all providers and as appropriate, 24 hours a day. *Patient care management* refers to all of the activities related to a patient's management. *Patient care support* relates to facility management of resources, including trend identification for quality improvement and utilization review and management purposes. *Billing and reimbursement* is the use of the record to provide justification for reimbursement for the care rendered, by describing the care in skilled terms.

The secondary purposes are education, regulation (compliance and accreditation), research, policymaking (allocating resources and planning), and industry (research and development).

Tables 1.3 and 1.4 list examples of the individual and institutional users of health records.[7] The patient identifiers are removed from all records used for purposes not directly related to patient care. In this way, the confidentiality of patient-identifiable information and the privacy of the individuals involved (both patients and providers) can be protected. However, the Health Insurance Portability and Accountability Act regulations requires specific patient permission for any primary or secondary use of the medical record as of April 2003.

Table 1.3
REPRESENTATIVE INDIVIDUAL USERS OF HEALTHCARE RECORDS

Patient Care Delivery (Providers)

Chaplains
Dental hygienists
Dentists
Dietitians
Laboratory technologists
Nurses
Occupational Therapists
Optometrists
Pharmacists
Physical Therapists
Physicians
Physician Assistants
Podiatrists
Psychologists
Radiology Technologists
Respiratory Therapists
Social Workers

Patient Care Delivery (Consumers)

Patients
Families

Patient Care Management and Support

Administrators
Financial Managers and Accountants
Quality Managers
Records Professionals
Risk Managers
Unit Clerks
Utilization Review Managers

Patient Care Reimbursement

Benefit Managers
Insurers (federal, state, and private)

Other

Accreditors
Government Policy Makers and Legislators
Lawyers
Healthcare Researchers and Clinical Investigators
Health Sciences Journalists and Editors

SOURCE: Dick, Steen, and Detmer 1997, p. 76.

Table 1.4
REPRESENTATIVE
INSTITUTIONAL
USERS OF HEALTH
RECORDS

Healthcare Delivery (Inpatient and Outpatient)

Alliances, associations, networks, and systems of providers
Ambulatory Surgery Centers
Donor banks (blood, tissue, organs)
Health Maintenance Organizations (HMOs)
Home Care Agencies
Hospices
Hospitals (General and Specialty)
Nursing Homes
Preferred Provider Organizations (PPOs)
Physicians offices (large and small group practices, individual practitioners)
Psychiatrics facilities
Public Health Departments
Substance Abuse Programs

Management and Review of Care

Medicare peer review organizations
Quality management companies
Risk management companies
Utilization review and utilization management companies

Reimbursement of Care

Business healthcare coalitions
Employers
Insurers (federal, state, and private)

Research

Disease registries
Health data organizations
Healthcare technology developers and manufacturers (equipment and device
    firms, pharmaceutical firms, and computer hardware and software vendors
    for patient record systems)
Research centers

Education

Allied Health professional schools and programs
Schools of medicine
Schools of nursing
Schools of public health

Accreditation

Accreditation organizations
Institutional licensure agencies
Professional licensure agencies

Policy Making

Federal government agencies
Local government agencies
State government agencies

SOURCE: Dick, Steen, Detmer 1997, p. 77.

Based on the primary and secondary purposes of the record, it is evident that a wide variety of individuals may require access to the record. Although terminology must be sophisticated and skilled enough to justify care, it must also be written in a manner that is clear and understood by other healthcare professionals, non-healthcare professionals, and others. Other users can be divided into individual and institutional users. Each user may use and need the information from the record for a different purpose. A chaplain offering spiritual guidance and comfort, uses information differently than a billing clerk, a third-party payer representative, physical therapist, or surveyor (i.e., Joint Commission on Accreditation of Healthcare Organizations [JCAHO], or Commission on Accreditation of Rehabilitation Facilities [CARF]). It is also becoming more common for the actual patient or patient representative, such as family, legal guardian, or healthcare surrogate, to take a greater interest in the care provided. With the exception of special regulations for psychiatric records, the Health Insurance Portability and Accountability Act of 1998 (HIPAA), ensures a patient or designated representative the right to see the record. For more information on HIPAA, see Chapter 7, Legal Issues in the Medical Record. The security, confidentiality, and privacy components of HIPAA were implemented in April 2003. The implications extend not only to current patients in any practice, but the maintenance of records as well. AHIMA recommends ten years for retention of records, JCAHO as determined by state law, CARF requires policies but specifies no time limits, and the National Committee on Quality Assurance (NCQA) does not specify.

The primary users of health records are patient care providers. However, many other individuals and organizations also use the information in health records. Managed care organizations, integrated healthcare delivery systems, regulatory and accreditation organizations, licensing bodies, educational organizations, third-party payers, and research facilities all use information that was originally collected to document patient care.

The Institute of Medicine broadly defines the users of health records as "those individuals who enter, verify, correct, analyze, or obtain information from the record, either directly or indirectly through an intermediary."[8] All users of health records influence clinical care in some way, but they use the information from health records for various reasons and in different ways. Some users (for example, nurses, physicians, and coding specialists) refer to the health records of specific patients as a part of their daily work. Many other users, however, never have direct access to the records of individual patients. Instead, they use clinical and demographic information.

As already noted, many individuals depend on the information in health records to perform their jobs. The individuals who provide direct patient care services include physicians, nurses, nurse practitioners, allied health professionals, and other clinical personnel. Allied health professionals include physician's assistants, physical therapists, respiratory therapists, occupational therapists, radiology technicians, and medical laboratory technicians. Other medical professionals, such as pharmacists, social workers, dietitians, psychologists, podiatrists, and chiropractors, also provide clinical services.

The services directly administered by patient care providers are documented directly into the patient's health record. Other service providers (for example, medical laboratory technicians) submit separate written reports that become part of individual health records.

Summary

The medical or client record is a comprehensive set of information that chronicles an episode of medically related care rendered to an individual. Medical record keeping or the process of health information management is necessary in healthcare for a variety of reasons. It should include all information related to a patient, expressed in terminology understood by all record users, both primary and secondary. Primary users of the record include those primarily involved in the care itself. Secondary users include most others. Regardless of the purpose the record serves, the content should be the same. By following general rules of medical record keeping and content, the physical therapist should be able to create documentation or a complete record (depending on setting) that will be universally understood and withstand scrutiny by any reader, for any purpose.

Chapter 1 Review Questions

1. What is the relationship between health information management and medical record keeping?

2. Whose responsibility is it to determine medical necessity for physical therapy?

3. The advent of what technology facilitated the ability for Medicare and others to track services rendered to beneficiaries?

4. Relative to documentation, why has physical therapy not been considered an essential medical service?

5. What is documentation according to the APTA Guide for Physical Therapist Practice?

6. Are the principles for documenting by manual entry different than for the electronic medical record? Defend your answer.

7. According to AHIMA, what are the primary purposes of the medical record?

8. Describe 5 secondary purposes of the medical record.

9. What does "user" mean in the context of the medical record? Give 5 examples and the purpose each would need to record for.

10. What is HIPAA and how is it relevant to health information management?

2

Record Organization and General Principles

General Principles

The management of medical records, including content and organization, should be consistent throughout the organization. There should be general rules for the content of all records and the professionals recording in the record. Additionally, the records should be organized so that individual pieces of information are easy to locate within the record as a whole. Therefore, all records in the same facility should be organized the same way.

Referral Information

Referral information—self-referred, physician referred or physician prescribed, consultation, or other—should be included in the patient's medical record. If the patient/client comes with a written order, that order becomes part of the record. If referred by verbal order, the person that took the order must transcribe it, consistent with state law. The transcription should also be followed up by a signed written referral, preferably an original rather than a fax. As of 2002, Medicare requires a copy of the physician referral/prescription in order to reimburse for services.

Storage

Records must be kept in locked, fireproof storage and accessible only to those directly involved with the patient/client. Electronic records must be password coded and screens must be shielded from public view. Security measures, such as firewalls, should also be in place.

Individual Charts/Folders

In facilities that use manual entry, there should be a single, hard copy "chart." If manila file folders are used, it is best practice to use a new folder for each new patient/client. If it is policy of the facility to reuse folders, all references on and in the folder to the prior patients/clients should be obliterated for privacy purposes.

Ink

For those organizations using manual entry, only ink should be used, preferably black or blue. In the recent past, black was generally expected and required. With the advent of improved copying systems, it can be difficult to discern an original from a copy. Therefore, from a legal perspective, some organizations have changed to blue ink. However, this is a decision for the organization or individual practitioner to make, and there should be consistency in color within the practice as outlined in a policy. Generally, black is still the ink color used for manual medical entries.

Legibility

All entries must be legible, not only to the writer, but to anyone who may need or is entitled to record access. Illegibility may give the impression of carelessness and rushed efforts. For electronic records, consistent font style and size should be used. Some electronic systems allow manual entry. In these systems, entries must be legible.

Data Types

Although not applicable to individual entries, the record as whole, regardless of the setting, consists of four types of data: "(1) personal, (2) financial, (3) social, and (4) medical," whether manual or electronic.[9]

Errors in the Record

Entries cannot be physically removed, completely covered, or otherwise made illegible. If items that should have been entered are recalled at any time following the documentation for a specific encounter, an addendum can be added. It must be placed in the next available space in the record and should include the time and date of entry. It should then state "Addendum to entry of _____."

If an error in spelling, location, or other minor error is made, a single line should be put through the incorrect entry. The correction should be made above the incorrect entry with the date and the initials of the person correcting beside it. Neither correction fluid (White Out) nor correction tape should be used in the medical record.

EXAMPLE

8/26/02 *ES*
18 y.o. male adm ~~8/25/02~~ with R femur fx.

Alterations to the medical record are considered fraudulent. Therefore, even if an incorrect entry is made on a new page and discovered, technically it should not be removed. Although this is current practice now, the privacy and confidentiality components of HIPAA may eventually require a change in this practice.

Additionally, do not leave blanks or skip lines and always enter information chronologically. Blanks may give the impression that information was forgotten and may leave opportunity for record alteration. Single lines can be drawn through or across multiple blank lines or spaces. However, in a system in which there are running chronological entries, the space that follows the final signature on an entry is not considered blank space and should not be lined out.

In electronic records, corrections must be made consistent with laws and acceptable practice.

Timeliness of Entry/Time of Session

Whether entries are dictated, manually written, or computer generated, they should be composed as close to the time of service delivery as possible, preferably at the time treatment is being rendered or immediately following. Timeliness of entry input saves time and ensures accuracy, as the PT does not have to "remember" what they did later. Additionally, if harm comes to the patient between PT visits, immediate documentation of patient status following treatment can protect the provider. If transcribed records cannot be obtained before the next patient visit, the provider should consider an alternate service that can deliver in a timely manner, or consider alternate forms of entry. This is especially relevant in the acute care setting with patients who are medically fragile or unstable. If another professional wanted to coordinate care, it could only be done if the records are entered in a timely manner. Discharge entries and summaries should also be completed in a timely manner for accuracy. Although good practice is to complete within 24 hours of discharge, it is up to the therapist to follow facility policies and procedures. There are regulations in place for some settings that do not require documentation for each visit. However, this may pose a problem to the provider for reimbursement purposes, continuity of care, blame if harm comes to the patient, and for liability purposes. According to the APTA, there should be an entry for every visit or encounter between patient and provider. Absence of an entry for any visit or encounter may result in denial of payment since there is no proof of the visit.

Spelling and Grammar

Although correct spelling and grammar would seem a given, carelessness does occur. The provider must correctly spell all words and write in a logical, coherent manner, as there are multiple uses for the record. Incorrect spelling and grammar may lead the reader to believe the care has been rendered with lack of skill. Professionals are expected to be able to spell. For electronic entry, some systems may have spell checks and grammar checks. If your system has these capabilities, it is recommended that they are used before finalizing entries.

Abbreviations

Only standard abbreviations and acronyms should be used. The dilemma in physical therapy is standardization. Refer to Appendix A for a list of some standard abbreviations. However, it is the organization's, facility's, or solo/independent practice PTs to have specific policies and procedures on using abbreviations. Individuals should not use self-developed abbreviations that are not universally understood. Abbreviations for specific PT treatments or interventions should only be used in conjunction with universally accepted Current Procedural Terminology (CPT® codes, universally required for billing) codes, to ensure categorical understanding. For example, other PTs or rehabilitation professionals may understand PNF for proprioceptive neuromuscular facilitation, but non-rehabilitation professionals would not know it is a form of therapeutic exercise. Additionally, if abbreviations have multiple meanings, such as WFL: within functional limits or within full limits, the PT should provide a key on the form being used.

Accuracy

All documentation entries should match billing dates, attendance grids, and appointment book entries. In the content itself, the medical diagnosis should be the one established by the referring medical professional as appropriate. The PT diagnosis should be established by the PT by description, matching International Classification of Disease codes (ICD-9 code, see a sample of ICD-9 codes in Appendix D), and must match the patient complaints, problems identified during the assessment, the goals established (functionally oriented), the intervention selected, and the frequency and duration of care. Each entry should match the appropriate billing date. The codes entered for billing purposes should match the codes and/or verbiage indicated in the record. CPT coding terminology should describe the interventions categorically. The PT diagnosis may be functionally oriented and therefore may differ or correspond with the medical diagnosis. The onset date of the PT problem should be clearly indicated. Throughout the record, all information should match.

Physical therapy diagnosis is not the same as medical diagnosis, and is actually a determination of the primary problem for which the patient is receiving or skilled care. For states in which PTs are not legally authorized to diagnose, the description would be the PT problem. The Medicare 700 series forms specifically require differentiation between the medical diagnosis and the physical therapy or treatment problem/diagnosis (See Appendix B).

Careful attention should be paid to using the correct word for homonyms or words that sound the same but are spelled differently and have different meaning, such as gait and gate and their and there. Care should also be taken to avoid any other commonly confused terms or concepts, such as left and right.

Information should be presented in an organized manner and indicate functional goals attained by the patient/client in a linear progression. The appropriate forms, as determined by policy and procedure or external requirements such as third-party payers, should always be used.

Authentication and Completion

To ensure authenticity and as a means of illustrating completion, the medical record entry should be signed by the physical therapist or physical therapist assistant who writes it. With dictated entries, the individual who dictated should read the entry when it is returned, then follow the other applicable rules regarding error correction, and sign. Original signatures are required with manual entry or dictation. Recently, electronic signature has been deemed legally acceptable in electronic records and faxed documents. Signature stamps, however, are not acceptable.

A legible signature should appear with every entry. If the entry spans multiple pages, it should appear on each page with continuation indicated. The signature should be the provider's full name and appropriate professional designation (i.e., PT or PTA) and should be signed the same way each time. It is recommended that the individuals' medical license number accompany the signature.

EXAMPLE

Susan Smith, PT, 0001977

Depending on state, national, local laws or accreditation requirements, student physical therapists and recent graduates with temporary licenses may require counter-signature or co-signature for authentication by the supervising licensed physical therapist. According to Roach, "The purpose of countersignatures is to require a professional to review, and if appropriate, indicate approval of action taken by another practitioner. Usually, the person countersigning a record entry is more experienced or has received a higher level of training than the person who made the original entry. In any case, the person required to countersign should be the individual who has the authority to evaluate the entry."[10]

EXAMPLE

Kevin Johnson, SPT
Susan Smith, PT 0001977

Courtesy

The record is not the place for complaints, criticism, blame, anger, arguments, or expressions of frustration with other healthcare team members. The tone of the entries should be as neutral as possible. If multiple attempts have been made by the therapist to contact a physician or another professional and he or she has not responded, simply record the date and time the call was made. Let others pass judgment. Avoid underlining for emphasizing negatively toned entries, do not change from cursive to print or vice versa, and do not write larger in some parts of the entry than others or in capital letters. In electronic records, or if manually printing, avoid using all capital letters as capitals indicate anger.

Content Inclusion

Document all telephone calls, missed appointments, instructions given to the patient/client or caregiver, discussion with families, verbal orders from physicians (followed by signed written orders in approximately 2 hours), instructions to other health professionals, all communication about the patient/client, and all relevant session/encounter information.

All entries should be meaningful and as objective as possible, including primarily facts. Do not write just for the sake of writing. Avoid phrases and words that are meaningless or have multiple meanings. If tempted to use the adjective confused for example, it is better to describe the behaviors that led you to use the word.

EXAMPLE

Instead of pt. is confused, write: Pt. could not identify therapist nor where he was.

Avoid phrases such as "tolerated treatment well." Describe, instead, what the patient or client accomplished in terms of time and endurance, or another choice of objective descriptions. Avoid PT jargon or terms and phrases only understood by PTs. What is written will influence the reader's impression of your care. Anyone that needs access to the record for any reason must be able to understand what is written. In the case of reimbursement, lack of understanding by the third-party payer representative may result in initial denial of a claim.

Terminology should be descriptive so that treatment can be duplicated or a clear picture of the patient/client is painted. Descriptive documentation should include impairments and functional limitations, justifying care based on functional improvement.

Headings or Titles

Preprinted forms or electronic templates usually include section headings or titles. In addition to section titles or headings, the whole entry itself should be titled (i.e., Physical Therapy Evaluation, Physical Therapy Notes, Physical Therapy Progress Report, etc.). In sections where narrative, paragraph, or "free form" entries may be included, it is better to categorize information. Even when using SOAP (subjective, objective, assessment, plan) format, subheadings can be used to clarify and better organize data than just the S O A and P. If categories extend to more than one page, either the back of a page or a new page, there should be an indication that it is a continuation. All pages should be numbered and total number should be clear (i.e. 1/4, 2/4, 3/4, 4/4).

Verbal Orders

The person taking the order should transcribe the verbal orders. State law may dictate who may take and transcribe the order. The entry itself should include what the order is for, the time it was taken, how it was taken (i.e., phone, face-to-face, phone message), the prescribing individual's name, and the name of the person who entered it. Verbal orders require authentication usually within 24 to 48 hours by the prescribing professional, based on organizational or accreditation guidelines or requirements.

Illustrations or Pictures

Pictures or illustrations can be effective tools for entering information into the record. They can be drawn with ink and must be clearly labeled, dated, and signed in addition to the body of the entry. Preprinted pictures must be clearly labeled as well (See Figure 2.1 for an example of a body diagram that can be utilized for documentation purposes).

Objectivity

All entries should be as objective as possible, avoiding subjectivity and including facts. Personal opinion should be avoided. If a patient comes in smelling of alcohol, yelling obscenities, and staggering, avoid documenting that they are drunk by instead documenting your observations of their behavior. Drunkenness can only be established legally by blood alcohol levels. Indeed, other medical conditions such as ketoacidosis may mimic drunkenness or alcohol breath.

Provide only the behaviors or signs that you have observed or assessed. When entering statements made by the patient/client, use quotation marks. When entering quotes, be careful when taking statements out of context.

Economy of Verbiage

All notes should be as efficient as possible, using only those words that are absolutely necessary. Nonessential words, such as pronouns and other modifiers, can be omitted. The reader will know, once the patient is identified, that entries are about the patient,

Figure 2.1
THE PAIN CHART

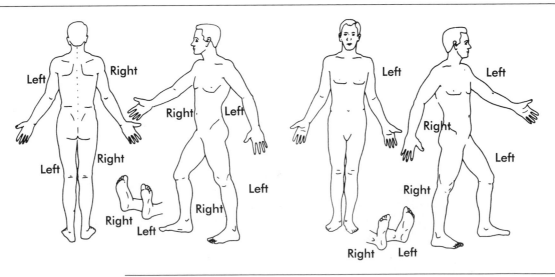

Instructions: Please use all of the figures to show exactly where all your pains are, and where they radiate to. Please be as precise and detailed as possible. Shade or draw with blue marker for pain. Use yellow marker for numbness and tingling; red marker for burning or hot areas; and green marker for cramping. Only the patient is to fill out this sheet. (Reproduced, with permission, from Melzack R. Pain Measurement and Assessment. *New York, Raven Press, 1983.)*

unless otherwise stated. When selecting words, if there are short alternatives, employ them, as long as the issue of "skilling" the note or care is not compromised. The use of commonly used or facility-approved symbols is also acceptable as a means of economizing on words. Bulleting or numbering can be used to present items in series. Electronic entries may have a selection of phrases based on function or diagnosis (See Appendix A abbreviations).

Denial Issues and Documentation

Although communicating the care of the patient is probably the most important purpose of documentation, the record is also used for reimbursement purposes. Although there are APTA guidelines regarding pro bono care, a practice or practitioner cannot survive on sole provision of intentional pro bono (unless supported by a grant or other source of funding). Nor can a practice or practitioner survive if charged services are not reimbursed. It is the responsibility of the professional providing care to ensure that the content of any entries in the patient/client record justify the intervention provided. The entries must, therefore, contain the information necessary to communicate with other practitioners involved in the care and ensure payment (as well as serve the other purposes of the medical record/documentation). When considering general principles of documentation and those specific to PT, discussion of the Office of the Inspector General (OIG) reports and identification of reasons for physical therapy denials in the Medicare system is warranted. These reports are accessible to the public and are available on the OIG web site (http://www.oig.dol.gov/), as well as the Centers for Medicare and Medicaid Services (CMS) web site (http://cms.hhs.gov/medlearn/therapy/oigrpts.pdf). The reasons include both technical errors and content errors that did not justify skilled PT intervention. Attention to the general principles of documentation can prevent denial for most of the elements cited and help the practitioner ensure appropriate content. The problems identified in the OIG audits, although performed on Medicare records, are universally applicable.

Common reasons for denials include:

- identifier omission
- incorrect form use
- incorrect information
- inadequate/imprecise
- illegibility
- good documentation in wrong place
- bad documentation in any place
- billing information did not match documentation of care
- goals did not match problems or diagnosis effectiveness of therapy services for patient's illness or injury (i.e., goals not achieved) not documented
- patient had achieved their restorative potential and were provided repetitive, non-skilled exercises (care exceeded date of goal achievement)
- patient did not require the care of a skilled therapist (either care was not skilled, maintenance too general, or the documentation did not indicate skill)
- loss of function or functional limitation not identified (problems were physiological impairment based)
- potential for significant improvement not identified (goals were not significant enough to justify care, or patient was too high level or too low level)
- need for skilled therapist not identified (improvement would have been made without therapeutic intervention)
- maintenance type therapies being provided (rote, repetitive treatment to maintain same level of function)

There are other common reasons for denial that will be described for the general knowledge of the therapist. Since authorization is frequently required in a managed care system for PT services, the following reasons for denial deserve attention. Although not considered documentation of care, they are part of the medical/client record. Authorization or pre-authorization is the permission of the third party payer or managed care organization (MCO) to provide a specified number of PT visits to a beneficiary. It usually includes total number of visits to an approved provider, based on a specific diagnosis with treatment authorized for a specific diagnosis for a specific body area or body part. As large third-party payers such as Blue Cross Blue Shield (BCBS) provide multiple insurance products, having provider status with one type or division does not automatically mean the therapist has provider status with another. For example, if a PT has a Medicare provider number through BCBS, it does not give the individual provider status with the Health Maintenance Organization (HMO) or Point of Service Plan (POS), unless the contract specifically stipulates otherwise. Pre-authorization or authorization does not necessarily ensure reimbursement. Documentation still has to support the necessity of skilled therapy services.

Reasons for denials based on authorization include:

- unauthorized treatment (where pre-authorization is required)
- unapproved provider (practice is not an approved provider for the payer)
- exceeded approval limit (exceeded pre-authorized number of visits in total, or goals were achieved in less than approved visits and treatment continued)
- treatment for other than "authorized" body area
- part of care justified by documentation, but not all (partial denial, either patient reached goals and there was continued care or only some of the documentation was skilled in nature)
- documentation did not support the need for skilled PT (not medically necessary)

Noncovered Conditions and Services

It is also the service provider's responsibility to be aware of medical conditions and services not covered by the third party payer. Regardless of the documentation, noncovered services will not be paid regardless of therapist efforts or goals. See Chapter 5, Coding and Documentation, for examples of Medicare noncovered services and conditions.

Summary

In 1996, federal auditors identified $23.2 million, or 14% Medicare overpayments. "Thirty-seven percent of improper payments were due to lack of medical necessity, such as payments for skilled physical therapy for patients with *no functional* diagnosis requiring physical therapy. . . . Incorrect coding was at the root of another 8.5% of the overpayments. Auditors checked codes by comparing the code with the documentation in the medical record to support that level of code."[11] Subsequent audits have yielded similar results.[12]

Results such as these have led to increasingly aggressive efforts by CMS to identify fraud and abuse in the Medicare system. All fiscal intermediaries and third-party payers are making the same efforts. With the advent of technology, audits and reviews can easily be performed to identify discrepancies.

Incorporating all of the general principles for documentation should help the therapist organize the record, record appropriate information, and get services reimbursed based on the documentation. The therapist should seek to write only what is relevant and necessary, in an objective manner, using verbiage that indicates skill, but is universally understood by all potential users of the medical record. By appreciating why payment for physical therapy services is denied, the therapist can reflect on documentation content guidelines and the importance of content adherence.

Chapter 2 Review Questions

1. How should manual and electronic records be stored?

2. Why is legibility imperative in the medical record?

3. Describe the types of data found in the medical record.

4. Explain how errors in the record should be corrected. Give 2 examples in different domains.

5. Explain the risks involved if entries into the record are not timely.

6. Why is the use of abbreviations in the record a potential problem for physical therapists?

7. Explain the concept of accuracy in the record.

8. What is co-signature? Provide an example of application in physical therapy documentation.

9. What does objectivity in the medical record mean?

10. What is the relationship between reimbursement and documentation? Give 6 examples of denial based on the documentation.

3

Application of Models for Organization and Guidelines for Content

Record Formats

There are a variety of record formats used by physical therapists and other professionals for manual entry or paper-based systems. (Note: the same formats may be used in the electronic or computerized record.) Categorically, they include source-oriented, problem-oriented, and integrated systems.

The *source-oriented medical record keeping system (SOMR)* has been commonly used in hospitals and skilled nursing facilities for decades. Each record or "chart" is divided into sections by profession or service given (i.e., physical therapy, nursing, medical, physician orders, laboratory, etc.). Patient problems are not separated and notes between caregivers are not integrated because they are "parallel" in nature. Entries in each section are usually in chronological order. It may be time consuming for the physical therapist to glean patient information from the SOMR because of this structure. Additionally, within each section, the methodology for recording information may be different for each discipline.

A component of the *problem-oriented medical record system (POMR),* the SOAP (subjective, objective, assessment, plan) note, is commonly used by physical therapists. Common use, however, should not be misunderstood to translate to the best or most effective or efficient for every situation. In an effort to improve patient record keeping, in 1958 Dr. Lawrence Reed of the University of Vermont, began exploring alternative types of record entries. The POMR, developed in 1969, focuses on a patient's specific problems in an integrated and coordinated manner between professionals. Weed's system includes the initial assessment, problem list, initial plan, progress notes, and discharge summary. All patient problems are included and numbered, active (current) and past, and all professionals involved in the patient's care contribute to the list. In the "pure" system, only one problem can be addressed on a SOAP progress note. Physician orders, not included in the initial plan, are cross-coded for relevance by number to the problems identified. Notes in the POMR are recorded in the SOAP or SOAPIER format. Weed offered categories to assist professionals in clarifying information.

S Subjective data (what the patient, family member, or significant other says the patient feels or is doing, *only as relevant to specific episode of care and problem.)*

AUTHOR'S NOTE

Beware of inclusion of statements that are irrelevant to care or, out of context, that may be misunderstood and result in denial of services.

O Objective data (what the professional observes, inspects or performs in a reproducible manner as relevant to function as possible and clearly presented)

A Assessment (summary of S & O with interpretation and professional judgment in order to justify care including progress toward goals if using SOAP only vs. SOAPIER)

P Plan (intervention plan)

I Implementation of plan

E Evaluation of the implemented plan

R Revision of the plan if necessary

The SOAP or SOAPIER entries may be supplemented by flow sheets for ongoing and frequent interventions. For the discharge summary, each problem identified needs a separate SOAP note by each professional providing intervention for the problem.

In order to adapt the SOAP note format to record-keeping regulations, an additional P for the patient problem, may be added before the S; PSOAP. In a hospital setting or skilled nursing facility (SNF), the record may be source oriented but the physical entry may be in POMR format, SOAP or PSOAP or SOAPIER. Another change in SOAP-type entries in the past decade is the introduction of functional outcomes reporting (FOR). In *Documenting Functional Outcomes* Abeln and Stewart furthered the concept of functional outcomes reporting or FOR, introduced by Swanson. This type of documenting stresses function and goals related to the same problem, and can be presented in SOAP format, the FOR format or narrative.

Dr. Weed's contribution to health or medical record keeping has, to date, passed the test of time. He envisioned "a future in which every patient will have a birth to death problem list on record for use by any hospital. This list, available through a central computer bank, would provide healthcare professionals with a patient's complete data base, anytime, anywhere."[13] Although Dr. Weed's vision has been a long time in coming, it is interesting to note that his vision is being realized. The recent experimental advent of implantable data chips is the realization of Dr. Weed's vision.

The third category of record keeping is the *integrated health record format*. All entries and forms by each discipline are arranged in chronological order without separation.

Individual Entry Formats

There are a variety of formats for individual entries, in addition to SOAP, including Problem, Status, and Plan (PSP); Problem, Status, Plan, and Functional Goals (PSPG); Data, Evaluation, Performance Goals (DEP); Functional Outcome Report (FOR); narrative; use of clinical tools; flow sheets/checklists; and illustrations. The latter three should be used more as supplements to the others than as stand-alone entries. In the past decade, documentation by exception and critical pathway documentation have also been introduced.

Problem Status Plan

P Patient problems and or medical diagnosis

S Patient/family/caretaker input as relevant and objective data

P Treatment plan/treatment rendered

Problem Status Plan and Functional Goals

P Patient problems and or medical diagnosis

S Patient/family/caretaker input as relevant and objective data

P Treatment plan/treatment rendered

G Functional goals/progress toward goals

Data Evaluation Performance Goals

D Patient/family/caretaker input as relevant and objective data

E Identification of patient problems, interpretation of data, treatment plan/treatment rendered

P Functional goals/progress toward goals

Functional Outcome Report (FOR)

The functional outcome report (FOR) includes the reason for referral, functional limitations (these differ from the American Physical Therapy Association [APTA] Nagi Model somewhat), physical therapy assessment, physical therapy problems, functional outcome goals/progress toward goals, treatment plan/treatment rendered, and rationale.

Narrative

Entries are made by category of intervention, possibly differentiated by terminology from Current Procedural Terminology Coding (CPT) in paragraph style format, objective intervention and patient response, progress toward goals, and plan or modifications to plan. There may be conclusions or assessments drawn, depending on the purpose of the entry (i.e., treatment vs. progress over time).

Clinical Tools

A variety of scales and indexes are commonly used in physical therapy. However, the use of tools must be coordinated with interventions and results external to the assessments or data gathered and entered onto the tool form. The information contained in the tool should always be summarized in a functional, objective manner in order to be meaningful to other professionals involved in care and any reader. Examples of clinical tools are the Berg Balance, Timed Get Up and Go, and the Folstein Mini Mental.

Functional Independence Measure (FIM)

Functional independence measure (FIM) is used to determine the severity of disability on a scale of 1 to 7. Developed by the University of Buffalo, the FIM scores are used to measure progress as a result of intervention, and is commonly used for inpatient rehabilitation. The Uniform Data Set administers the system. Fees are charged for participation in the system and analysis of the data for one organization compared to similar organizations in the system. FIM is functionally oriented, using variables such as transfer, toileting, and gait. The WeeFIM is the version of FIM used for pediatric application.

Focus on Therapeutic Outcomes, Inc. (FOTO)

The Focus on Therapeutic Outcomes, Inc. (FOTO) system is designed to measure outcomes of care in the outpatient setting. Like the FIM system, fees are charged for participation in the system and analysis of the data for your organization compared to similar organizations in the system.

Flowsheets and Checklists

Flowsheets and checklists may contain dates, treatments, attendance, or a variety of other activities. Generally, a check mark is used to mark a specific box for the care provided. Initials of the person who provided the care are preferable to discourage others from entering on the record. Flowsheet or checklist entries should be accompanied by notes to clarify entries and "skill" or rate the effectiveness of the intervention. Although functional, they should not be used as stand-alone forms. See Table 3.1 for a flowsheet example.

Table 3.1
FLOWSHEET EXAMPLE

TX:	8/26/03	8/27/03	8/28/03
Ther ex	*JfS*		
Gait Training	*JfS*		
Functional Training		*JfS*	
Home Instruction		*JfS*	

Supplemental entries by date:

8/26/03 "Pain at 3/10 during activity after last session." Able to inc. resistance from 5 to 8#'s for quad ext/flex, 30 reps. Demonstrated ability to ascend and descend 5 steps without use of handrails, no knee buckling. Steady improvement noted. *Jon f. Smith, PT, # 1234*

8/27/03

Critical Pathways/Clinical Pathways

Within each patient's therapy plan, target processes and sequences of care, known as critical or clinical pathways, are determined upon the initial visit or diagnosis and generally follow a precise timeline. The pathways are generally experientially or evidence based, and may be used to replace traditional forms of documentation since they require only a signature and date when a goal is achieved on a preprinted pathway form. The term critical pathway relates to the original pathways developed in acute care for "critically ill" patients. Clinical pathways are more applicable in rehabilitation for patients not "critically" ill. See Table 3.2 for a clinical pathway example.

Documentation by Exception

The documentation by exception style of record keeping consists of using anticipated or typical treatments and goals that are pre-established and available on preprinted forms in manual entry systems. The only entries required would be variations from the established "norms." In electronic or computerized systems, the user enters the initial diagnosis and the treatment information appears in a retrievable file in a data bank. This method is not recommended because it does not allow for entry of specific patient information and is often too generalized.

Principles Specific to Physical Therapy

Documentation content can be organized and simplified with the use of models. Models are frequently used in industry and theoretical sciences to make categorization of information easier to study, organize, apply, and discuss. The APTA provides models in the *Guide to Physical Therapist Practice*. The information in the Guide is presented using a Nagi-based disablement model and the Clinical Decision-Making Model (CDMM) see Figure 3.1. Using the disablement model and the CDMM can help therapists organize their examination (tests and measures), evaluation, interventions, and all record-keeping documentation.

Exclusive of the models, guidelines for documentation were first established for Medicare by the Healthcare Finance Administration (HCFA, now Center for Medicare and Medicaid, CMS). Initially the guidelines were used by the Medicare fiscal intermediaries (FIs) or carriers, to verify provision of services to beneficiaries by physicians. The guidelines were not, however, used extensively until the 1970s. By

Table 3.2
CLINICAL PATHWAY EXAMPLE

Medical Diagnosis: _____

PT Diagnosis: _____

Weight Bearing Status: _____ RLE _____ LLE

PT Name: Print: _____ Signature: _____ Initials: _____
PT Name: Print: _____ Signature: _____ Initials: _____
PT Name: Print: _____ Signature: _____ Initials: _____
PT Name: Print: _____ Signature: _____ Initials: _____
PT Name: Print: _____ Signature: _____ Initials: _____

IEP:

Post-op day achieved	Quad sets, ankle pumps	Able to recall precautions	LTD Asst bed mob	I bed mobility	I sit <> supine	Min Asst Sit <> stand	Min Asst Gait with walker, 25	Sup standing with device	Pain level with movement
1	JFS	JFS							10/10
2			JFS	JFS	JFS	JFS			9/10
3					JFS	JFS			7/10
4							JFS	JFS	6/10
5									

Discharge status:

Indicate if status different from that above:

Supplemental entries as indicated:

Figure 3.1
PHYSICAL THERAPY DECISION-MAKING MODEL

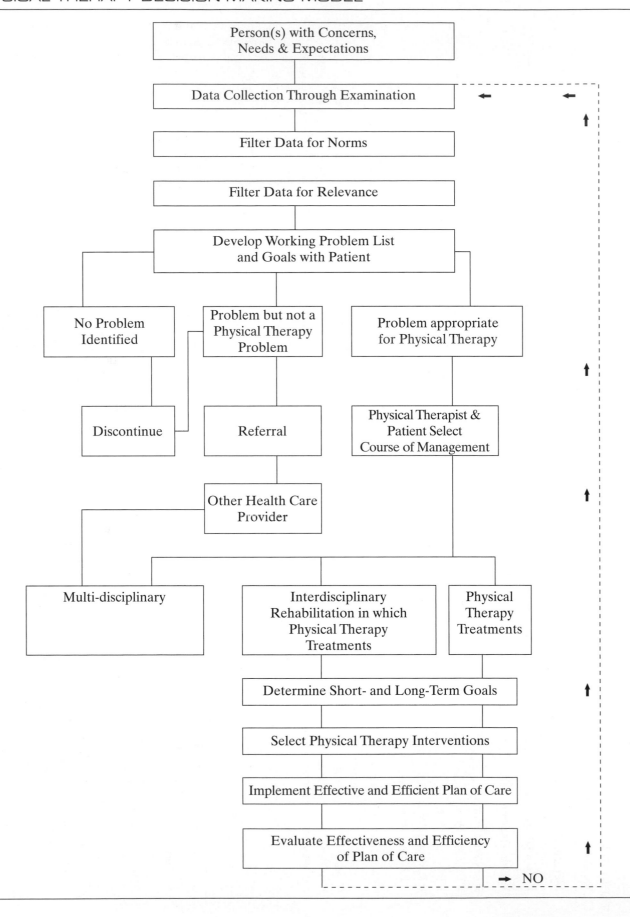

Figure 3.1
PHYSICAL THERAPY DECISION-MAKING MODEL

the 1970s, computers could track adherence and costs to the system, which began to grow exponentially. When non-Medicare providers (also known as carriers or third-party payers) gained access to technology and the revelation that they too could track provision of care, documentation for non-Medicare beneficiaries had to undergo the same scrutiny. Though somewhat general in nature, there is standard information required by Medicare. Many of the guidelines were written into Medicare manuals in the 1970s and 1980s, but it was not until a decade later that Medicare attempted to standardize forms or formats for reimbursement.

It should be noted that the information required in Medicare documentation is very similar to that recommended in the APTA *Guidelines for Physical Therapy Documentation*.[14] The Medicare documentation guidelines can be obtained on the Internet by accessing Medicare provider manuals at www.cms.gov.

The Disablement Model

As early as the 1970s, disablement models were developed with the following help of sociologist Saad Nagi to categorize the impact of medical conditions on function for The World Health Organization (WHO). WHO, part of a component organization of the United Nations, which also developed the International Classification of Diseases (ICD–9), developed an alternative model in 1980, the International Classification of Diseases, Impairments, Disabilities, and Handicaps. The National Center for Rehabilitation and Research developed a similar model in 1992. See Table 3.3 for the disablement models.

The *Guide to Physical Therapist Practice* uses the Nagi framework as the theoretical basis for its terminology. Familiarity with the model should help the PT in conceptualiz-

Table 3.3
DISABLEMENT MODELS

	NAGI	WHO	National Center for Rehabilitation and Research
Categorization of condition	Active Pathology: Interruption or interference with normal processes and efforts of the organism to regain normal state	Disease: The intrinsic pathology or disorder	Pathophysiology: Interruption with normal physiological developmental processes or structures
Impairment	Anatomical, physiological, mental, emotional abnormalities, or loss	Loss or abnormality of psychological, physiological, or anatomical structure or function at organ level	Loss or abnormality of cognitive, emotional, physiological, or anatomical structure or function
Activities	Functional limitation: limitation in performance at the level of the whole person	Disability: Restriction or lack of ability to perform an activity in normal manner	Functional limitation: Restriction or lack of ability to perform in action in the manner or range consistent with the purpose of an organ system
End state	Disability: Limitation in performance of socially defined roles and tasks within a social, cultural, and physical environment	Handicap: Disadvantage as a result of impairment or disability that limits or prevents fulfillment of a normal role depending on age, gender, or sociocultural factors for the person	Societal limitation: Restriction attributable to social policy or barriers that limit fulfillment of roles

ing and actualizing documentation of care, as all components should be addressed in the medical or client record. There are four categories in the model: pathology or pathophysiology, impairment, functional limitation, and disability. Pathology or pathophysiology is a situation in which an injury is caused by a disorder, condition, or disease. Impairment is the physiologic or system problem itself (i.e., integument, cardiopulmonary or neuromuscular, psychological, or anatomical problem). Functional limitation is activity limitation that occurs as a result of the impact of the impairments on a physical "action, task, or activity in an efficient, typically expected, or competent manner."[15] Disability is the inability to perform expected self-care, leisure, work, community, and social roles.

By addressing all four elements of the disablement model, the PT should be able to appropriately address patient/client needs and problems, regardless of the format the PT selects to enter the information (i.e., SOAP or narrative). The functional goals of the episode of care should be based on resolution or management of the impairments as they relate to function, decrease or eliminate functional limitations and decrease or eliminate disabilities. The record should not, however, ever reflect concentration on physiologic impairment or resolution of impairments, unless a clear relationship is established between the impairment and its impact on functional improvement. Patient problems can be summarized in the Initial Examination/Evaluation by using the classification headings, which better articulate the treatment goal. *If specifics have already been stated in the body of the document,* deficits can be summarized as follow.

EXAMPLE

Impairments	Functional limitations	Disabilities
• Limited bilateral knee flexion limited to 30°/135°	• Unable to climb stairs in home • Unable to sit at table or desk • Unable to squat	• Unable to work as a driver

The above is characteristic of the functional reporting model. With appropriate form development and organization, goals and anticipated dates can be added as columns to clearly relate impairments to functional limitations and disabilities.

Another application of the disablement model as a tool to facilitate thinking and organization of record content is the Clinical Decision-Making Model (Figure 3.1). The Clinical Decision-Making Model (CDMM) helps the therapist organize the patient/client management process from initial visit through discharge, using the same documentation process throughout. Recording of the information gained by history and interview and various tests and measures, should assist in filtering the data for relevance to PT management. Clearly documenting problem summaries and setting realistic functional goals should result in a well-constructed initial evaluation document.

The *Guide to Physical Therapist Practice* suggests six components for patient/client management that lead to "optimal outcomes:"

Diagnosis

↕

Evaluation

↕

Examination

↕

Prognosis

↕

Intervention

↕

Outcomes

The specific elements in the six components can be correlated to the categories of information that should be included in the written record as follows.

Diagnosis

Based on the examination results and clinical judgment, the therapist determines the PT diagnosis or problem and correlates it with the appropriate functional ICD-9 code or ICD-10 (if in use at time). The initial examination/evaluation should also include the physician's referring diagnosis. However, the therapist should beware of medical diagnoses that absolutely do not match actual treatment diagnoses, as they will interfere with reimbursement.

EXAMPLE

Medical Diagnosis: fractured humerus   ICD-9: 812.12 (closed, unspecified)

                                                              812.30 (open)

This may be sufficient if the referral was for treatment of the healing humerus or the individual had become dependent in self-care. However, if the referral was because the patient/client had lost gait functionality because of prior walker use, then the PT diagnosis or problem should be different:

EXAMPLE

PT diagnosis: gait abnormality   ICD-9: 781.2

A diagnosis that does not match the problems, interventions, or goals identified will result in denial of the claim.

Generally, an acute medical event such as the onset of a cerebrovascular accident (CVA), fracture, multiple trauma or multisystem illness, or presence of co-morbidities or complex medical condition will justify, with appropriate documentation, skilled physical therapy.

Examination

Information and data obtained during the examination process (tests and measures), leads the therapist to clinical judgments, including appropriate systems, screening, and more specific tests and measures to determine the patient/client needs. The specific tests and measures are usually categorized on a "form" entitled PT Evaluation with varying formats. For certain Medicare venues such as a Skilled Nursing Facility (SNF) or a Certified Outpatient Rehabilitation Facility (CORF), the results of the initial examination and evaluation are entered into the CMS 700 form (See Appendix B), or a self-designed form that includes the same information.

Evaluation

Based on information and data collected, the therapist makes clinical judgments regarding patient care, including identification of the PT problem or diagnosis and potential need for consultation or referral. According to the APTA *Guidelines for Documentation,* this stage is called the Initial Examination and Evaluation/Consultation. In total, this entry should answer the following questions:

1. Who is the patient?

   Demographics, medical history, social history, prior or concurrent services (avoid duplication), onset

2. Where is the patient functionally?

   Causative impairments, functional limitations, disabilities

3. What is/are the primary problems the patient has?

   System tests and measures, impairments, medical/social/psych problems that may impact care

4. What is the applicable PT diagnosis?

   The primary problem that will be addressed correlated to the appropriate ICD-9 code

5. Can the problems be impacted by PT intervention?

   Identification of effective and efficient intervention for the problem(s)

6. If yes, which will be addressed during this episode of care?

   Identification of the problem(s) that will be addressed in the plan of care

7. If no, what will the disposition be?

   If not accepting the individual for care, identify reason: lack of expertise in area of problem, has other problems that need referral in addition to those for PT, problems identified are not within scope of PT

Prognosis

According to the *Guide to Physical Therapy Practice,* the prognosis is included in the Initial Examination/Evaluation document, including the plan of care (interventions), goals or level of function anticipated as a result of the therapeutic intervention, and frequency and duration of treatment. Contents for the plan of care are outlined by CMS for Medicare beneficiaries. However, they can be applied to all settings and carriers. The prognosis also includes the individual's rehabilitation potential, which is relevant to the PT goals and prior level of function. If an individual is accepted for care, the rehabilitation potential should be at most good. Excellent may appear to indicate to the reader that the individual may not need services. If the PT chooses fair, it may be acceptable assuming the patient is too ill to make any other determination at the time.

Intervention

These are the specific skilled PT treatments and methods used to impact the patient's problems and achieve goals established by the PT in conjunction with the patient/client. The treatments should be described with terminology that matches Current Procedural Terminology (CPT), the AMA billing codes or HCPCS. (Refer to Chapter 5)

Outcomes Assessment

This phase of treatment occurs when the results of the interventions or treatments are evaluated. The *Guide to Physical Therapy Practice* includes the re-examination of the patient/client with intervention to determine if changes or modifications are needed in the interventions. If the patient is not demonstrating progress towards the desired outcomes or achieving the anticipated results from the interventions or treatment at any point in time, re-evaluation of treatment options is necessary. Possible adjustments in treatment include changing intervention and determination of change in medical status necessitating referral back to the physician or initial referral in states with direct access. The outcome or progress level during care must be clearly indicated in the documentation. If some or all of the goals are not achieved, the reasons for lack of accomplishment must be included. These outcomes must also reflect back to the initial goals and modifications during the episode of care.

Summary

There are three basic formats for medical/client record organization: the SOMR, POMR, and integrated systems. Of the three, the SOMR, the system that divides the record by service or discipline, is the most common. Each service, however, may choose within the SOMR to make their entries in the "model" of their choice. The most common entry formats for PT are a SOAP and narrative, for ongoing entries, with flowsheets and checklists for intervention parameters. A variety of customized formats, often self-designed, are used for initial examination/evaluation and discharge summaries and disposition.

In the *Guide to Physical Therapist Practice,* the APTA purports using the Nagi Disablement Model to help organize patient/client care and the documentation. In the model, information is divided into pathology, impairment, functional limitation, and disability. The Guide identifies six elements that must be included in the record: the PT diagnosis or problem (as well as the medical as applicable), examination, evaluation, prognosis, intervention (continuation of care), and outcomes assessment (summation of episode of care). Application of the concepts presented in the *Guide to Physical Therapist Practice* and the Clinical Decision-Making Model can assist the PT is completing appropriate documentation.

Chapter 3 Review Questions

1. What are the basic types of medical record organization? Compare and contrast these types.

2. Explain what goes in each section of the SOAP formatted note. What is the difference between the SOAP and SOAPIER?

3. Give examples of three types of individual entry formats. Compare and contrast each format.

4. What is your opinion regarding the popularity of the SOAP format?

5. What is a clinical tool and its relevance to documentation? Give two examples.

6. Why is it not prudent to use a checklist or flowsheet without additional narrative or written entries?

7. Explain what a disablement model is. Which model is used by the APTA in the *Guide to Physical Therapist Practice?*

8. Explain the categories in the disablement model employed in the *Guide to Physical Therapist Practice.* Include examples for each category.

9. Give an example of an impairment, the resulting functional problem, and possible disability.

10. Compare and contrast the medical diagnosis and the physical therapy diagnosis (physical therapy problem).

11. What is the difference between the initial examination and the evaluation?

CHAPTER

4 Component Requirements

General Documentation Requirements

HCFA Medicare regulations were the first to delineate documentation requirements for physical therapists (PTs). Although there are some differences depending on setting and type of organization, there are basic requirements for all PT services: physician order (except for direct access, although may be required for third party reimbursement), evaluation, plan of care, certification of the plan of care (POC), ongoing documentation of care, reevaluation, and discharge summary. There are also states, such as Florida, that include documentation requirements in the practice act, although they are similar to those required by Medicare. In the last decade, the American Physical Therapy Association (APTA) has developed guidelines for documentation that are similar to the Medicare guidelines (See Table 4.1). It is interesting to note that the Medicare program does not require its providers to abide by the same documentation requirements for non-Medicare patients. However, in the states in which documentation requirements are included in the laws, and for those therapists that follow APTA guidelines, the requirements are very similar.

Because these documentation elements are generic and widely used, therapists should attempt to use them consistently, regardless of the third-party payer or payment system. The only documentation differences between patients should be the type of goal (i.e., pediatrics vs. geriatrics) or form requirements for billing (i.e., CMS 1500 vs. CMS 700 or 701). Durable medical equipment, such as orthotics or wheelchairs, may require not only the standard documentation to identify need, but additional supporting letters from the therapist and/or physician, or state-specific forms, such as for Florida Medicaid wheelchairs.

Initial Examination or Evaluation

The APTA includes four categories of content: general guidelines, initial examination and evaluation/consultation, continuation of care, and summation of the episode of care. Practitioners may be more familiar with the colloquial terms of initial evaluation, daily/weekly notes, progress notes/reports, and discharge reports or summaries.

What is important for each, regardless of the name, is the content. The initial report sets the tone for the record and should clearly establish the need for skilled therapy. Many of the elements included are repeated in the discharge summary to determine if indeed the care rendered matches the initial problems and plan. All data should be communicated as objectively as possible to allow for objective goal setting and justification of care. The categories from "Referral through Precautions" to "Reason for Skill through Authentication" should be included in all records. The therapist will have to make decisions regarding which baseline tests and measures should be included based on the patient/client primary complaint(s).

Table 4.1 MEDICARE (CMS) AND APTA GUIDELINES FOR DOCUMENTATION	**Medicare** (requires some forms or similar format and content)	**APTA: Guide for Documentation** (provider choice of format)
	Physician's order (prescription)	Referral or referral mechanism
	Evaluation	Initial Examination/Evaluation
		History
	Identification of objective losses by system	Systems review
		Tests & measures
		Evaluation: judgment
		PT diagnosis
	Prognosis	Prognosis
		Pt./client involvement in goals
		Measurable goals related to Impairment, Functional
	Plan of care	Limitations, Disabilities
		Plan of care
		Authentication
	Ongoing documentation of interventions	Continuation of care
		Every visit or encounter
	Reevaluation/Recertification	Reexamination
	Discharge	Summation of episode of care

Initial Visit

For record authenticity purposes, it is preferable to include as much information as possible in the record at the initial visit. In some situations, some of the tests and measures may have to be completed on subsequent visit(s), although as much as possible should be completed so an initial plan can be developed.

Content of Initial Visit Documentation
Referral Information. The two types of referrals in PT are self-referred and physician referred. If the patient is physician referred, the diagnosis(es) and treatment requested must be included on the prescription according to the 2002 Medicare guidelines.

Signed Consent. Signed acknowledgement of organization HIPAA policies. Required to treat by patient/client, legal guardian, or parent

Patient/Client Identification Information. Full name, gender, date of birth, and language spoken: primary and secondary

Start of Care Date (SOC). Date of the initial examination/evaluation for the episode of care

Medical Diagnosis. If physician referred or if known by patient

Physical Therapy Diagnosis. PT diagnosis or primary PT problem with recent onset date. If an injury, list the mechanism of it. If a chronic condition, list date of acute or recent exacerbation.

Medical History. Include co-morbidities (may be summarized if on separate intake form completed by patient/client with only relevant information summarized in the evaluation) and medications, as they may impact physical therapy, recent hospitalizations, circumstances regarding onset.

Related Medical Testing Results. As available to PT.

Patient/Client/Family Therapy Goals. Goals determined based on examination results and needs of patient/client/family

Prior Functional Level. This should include mobility (home and community); work, school, leisure, and self-care (ADL [activities of daily living], IADL [instrumental activities of daily living]); family care responsibilities/child care/elder care

Social History/Support. Handedness: right/left; employment income source, school, leisure; family status; living arrangements (type of dwelling, presence or absence of stairs, location of bedrooms and bath); support system

Precautions/Contraindications/Barriers. Precautions may relate to medical conditions as with cardiac precautions, surgical as in total hip precautions, weight bearing, or other. Contraindications would indicate that some procedure should not be performed for a specific reason (i.e., electrical stimulation to a body area close to a non-shielded pacemaker), or ultrasound use over a non-healed fracture site. Barriers may include such things as physical barriers in a living environment, illiteracy, language, or regular transportation.

Baseline Data from Tests and Measures

- Activities of daily living (instrumental and functional, compare to prior level of function);
- Activity tolerance/Endurance;
- Balance;
- Cardiovascular/pulmonary;
- Cognition;
- Coordination;
- Gait;
- General integrity;
- Hearing;
- Joint integrity;
- Mobility (bed, wheelchair);
- Motor control/movement patterns (gross and fine motor skills);
- Muscle performance/strength;
- Musculoskeletal;
- Neuromuscular/neuromotor development;
- Pain (measurable scale of 0/10 to 10/10, specifying body part and pain at rest and activity);
- Posture;
- Range of motion: active vs. passive; vs. active assistive;
- Reflexes;
- Sensory/proprioception;
- Systems review (as relevant to problem for specific episode of care);
- Tone;
- Transfers/transitional movement;

- Vascular: capillary refill, skin temperature/condition, edema, extremity hair patterns, nails;
- Vision;
- Vital signs: radial pulse (other peripheral as applicable, blood pressure, respiration rate, breathing pattern) before, during, and after;
- Integument: Wounds/ulcerations/any abnormalities or potential areas of concern;
- Functional deficits

Device Use. Orthotics; prosthetics; assistive gait devices; communication devices (i.e., augmentative communication devices, communication boards, speech, hearing aids, glasses, electrolarynx [external]

Note: Passy-Muir valves have replaced the need for electrolarynx in some cases in recent years.

Results of any special tests.

Architectural/Safety Considerations. The physical considerations of the home, work, school, and other environments/buildings including access, presence of stairs, elevators, ramps, bathrooms, door widths, bathroom accessibility, and so on. Safety relates to the patient/client's ability to function safely in an environment based on their abilities.

Reason for Skilled Care, Assessment/Professional Judgment.

Problem Summary. The PT medical record should also include a summary of deficits identified in baseline data, preferably delineating the relationship between impairments and the functional limitations and disabilities, but avoiding physiological impairment focus. There is a difference in functional outcome reporting versus the *Guide to Physical Therapist Practice* regarding impairment and functional limitation. In the Nagi disablement model, which is used in the guide, gait is considered an impairment. Gait in different environments and levels of quality, speed, and functional purposes are considered functional limitations. For Medicare purposes, concentration should be on essential functional activities (EFA) as much as possible, based on the setting in which the patient/client is being treated. For example, home health would concentrate on EFA in the home. Once the progression is made to outpatient, essential activities would expand into the environment outside the home and appropriate safe function.

Plan of Care (POC).

The PT plan of care (POC) should include specific planned interventions using CPT or HCPCS terminology, including patient/caregiver instruction and a statement regarding patient/family involvement in goal setting. The POC should list the frequency and duration of the treatment and include all short- and long-term goals (time defined, functionally oriented). Rehabilitation potential for achievement of goals/prognosis should also be included along with a statement of the medical necessity or need for skilled PT.

AUTHOR'S NOTE

Medicare providers may have a separate document entitled POC since physician signature is required.

Authentication. Authentication consists of the signature of the both the PT and the referring physician (for a Medicare POC) with attestation of the need for skilled PT and agreement with the POC.

According to the Medicare Carrier Manual, the following must be included:

a. Identification of the physician's order for physical therapy

b. Indication that the patient is under the care of a physician or optometrist for the presenting diagnosis

c. Indication of the potential prognosis for restoration of functions in a reasonable and generally predictable period of time

d. Patient identification information

e. Precautions/contraindications/barriers

All providers billing for physical therapy services are required to maintain an established plan of treatment as a permanent part of the patient's clinical record. The plan must be established before the treatment is begun. The physician or optometrist must see the patient at least every 30 days during the course of therapy. The physician or optometrist must review, initial, and date the plan of treatment at least every 30 days.

AUTHOR'S NOTE

This is applicable for Part B in out-patient venues such as Skilled Nursing Facilities, Rehabilitation Agencies, home health, and independent practitioners. For Certified Outpatient Facilities (CORF) it is 60 days for the initial POC (Plan Of Care), then every 30 days.

The plan must be kept on file in the physician or optometrist's office and available for carrier review if requested.

A physical therapy plan of treatment must include the type, amount, frequency, and duration of the services that are to be furnished and indicate the diagnosis and anticipated goals. Any changes in the treatment plan must be made in writing and signed by the physician or optometrist.

Medical record documentation maintained by the ordering/referring physician or optometrist must clearly indicate the medical necessity of each physical therapy modality covered by the Medicare program.

The physician, optometrist and/or therapist *must document the patient's functional limitations in terms that are objective and measurable.* Documentation must show objective loss of joint motion, strength, or mobility (i.e., degrees of motion, strength grades, levels of assistance.)

All claims submitted with an unlisted service or procedure must be accompanied by documentation that describes the service, supports medical necessity, and the rationale for using the treatment modality.

The Medicare guidelines, available at www.cms.gov in the provider manuals and on the First Coast of Florida Web site, state the following relative to the POC:

Services must be furnished under a plan of treatment that has been written and developed by the physician caring for the patient. The plan must be established prior to the initiation of treatment, must be signed by the physician, and must be incorporated into the physician's permanent record for the patient. The services provided must relate directly to the written treatment regimen.

The plan of care must contain the following information:

1. Patient's diagnoses that require physical therapy;

2. The patient's significant past history;

3. Related physician orders;

4. Therapy goals and potential for achievement;

5. Any contraindications;

6. Patient's awareness and understanding of diagnoses, prognosis, treatment goals; and

7. When appropriate, the summary of treatment provided and results achieved during previous periods of physical therapy services.

2206.3 <u>Outpatient Physical Therapy or Speech Pathology Services Furnished Under Plan</u>—Outpatient physical therapy or speech pathology services are furnished under a plan established and periodically reviewed by a physician. The plan is established (that is, reduced to writing either by the physician who makes the plan available to the clinic or by the clinic personnel when they make a written record of the physician's oral order) before treatment is begun. The plan is promptly signed by the ordering physician and incorporated into the clinic's permanent record for the patient.

The plan relates the type, amount, frequency, and duration of the physical therapy that are to be furnished to the patient and indicates the diagnosis and anticipated goals. Changes are made in writing and signed by the physician, a qualified physical therapist (in the case of physical therapy), a qualified speech pathologist (in the case of speech pathology services), a registered professional nurse, or physician on the staff of the clinic pursuant to the attending physician's oral orders.

Outpatient physical therapy may be furnished under a written plan of treatment established by the qualified physical therapist providing such physical therapy services as long as the physician periodically reviews the plan.

Physical therapy services are to be furnished in accordance with the plan of care established by the physician responsible for the patient's care and may not be altered in type, amount, or duration by the therapist (except in the case of an adverse reaction to a specific treatment).

2206.1 <u>Physician's Certification and Recertification.</u>
A. <u>Content of Physician's Certification.</u>—Medicare does not pay for outpatient physical therapy unless a physician certifies that:

- The services are or were required by the patient.

- A plan for furnishing such services is or was established and periodically reviewed by the physician. . . . A plan of treatment for outpatient physical therapy services is established by either the physician or the qualified physical therapist providing such services. However, a plan established by a physical therapist must be periodically reviewed by the physician . . . (See §2206.3.)

The outpatient physical therapy services are or were furnished while the patient was under the care of a physician. (See §2206.2.)

Since the certification is closely associated with the plan of treatment, the same physician who established or reviews the plan of treatment, must certify the necessity for services. Obtain certification at the time the plan of treatment is established or as soon thereafter as possible.

Recertification Documentation

When outpatient physical therapy services are continued under the same plan of treatment for a period of time, the physician must recertify at intervals of at least once every 30 days that there is a continuing need for such services and estimate how long services are needed. Obtain the recertification at the time the plan of treatment is reviewed since the same interval (at least once every 30 days) is required for the review of the plan. The physician who reviews the plan of treatment signs the recertifications. The form of the recertification and the manner of obtaining timely recertification is the responsibility of the individual clinic.

AUTHOR'S NOTE

For Certified Outpatient Rehabilitation Facilities (CORF), the requirement for recertification is every 60 days for the initial 60. It is then every 30 days. All other outpatient physical therapy, skilled nursing, and home health requires 30 days. The requirements for out-patient coverage by Medicare are essentially the same for all settings. For non-Medicare, the Medicare guidelines can be applied by provider choice.

Coverage and
Limitations

Medicare Guidelines, Section 2206.2 B: Method and Disposition of Certifications. There is no requirement that the certification or recertification be entered on any specific form or handled in any specific way as long as you can determine, where necessary, that the certification and recertification requirements are met. The certification by the physician is retained by the clinic, and the clinic certifies on the billing form that the requisite certifications and recertifications have been made by the physician and are on file in the clinic when it forwards the request for payment to you.

Medicare Guidelines, Section 2206.2 C: Delayed Certification. The clinic must obtain certifications and recertifications as promptly as possible. Payment is not made unless the necessary certifications are secured. In addition to complying with the usual content requirements, delayed certifications and recertifications are to include an explanation for the delay and any other evidence the clinic considers necessary in the case. The format of delayed certifications and recertifications and the method by which they are obtained is left to the clinic.

Medicare guidelines further state that it is expected that therapy services be performed as indicated by current medical literature and/or standards of practice. When services are performed in excess of established parameters, they may be subject to review for medical necessity. This concept should guide the therapist in all entries and treatments.

Documentation of Continuation of Care

According to the Medicare regulations, "The office/progress note must contain necessary and sufficient information, which indicates the services were actually provided and were reasonable and necessary to treat the patient's condition." The categories described in the APTA guidelines include "Documentation of intervention or services provided and current patient/client status, and Documentation of Reexamination."[16] It is the therapist's or organization's responsibility to determine the format in which the information should be included.

The APTA guidelines do not describe types of entries, but rather content. However, as PTs and PTAs tend to describe types of entries, following are descriptions of entry types, but not descriptions of format. Again, that is the decision of the therapist.

Types of Entries

APTA: Continuum of Care. Daily Note/Treatment Note (format of choice)

- Where rendered and how pt. arrived
- Characteristics/Content: Brief entries that contain basic identification. If continuous on a page, this is only needed at the top of each page.
- Patient/client statement of response to treatment for that session and since previous
- Specific interventions where applied, i.e., lower extremity.
- Equipment issued, if any
- Response to intervention at that visit (+ or −)
- Instructions given/communication and if pt. was accompanied and who it was.
- Brief statement of overall functional progress, not necessarily addressing all goals (as in progress reports)
- Additions/deletions of treatments
- Statement regarding plan for next visit
- Authentication

AUTHOR'S NOTE

A progress note would include the same information as a treatment note in addition to a statement of progress relative to the initial or interim goals established. It is usually longer as it relates to a longer period of time, i.e., a week, multiple weeks.

APTA Continuum of Care, Forms/Checklists: Forms include space for consecutive days/sessions, modalities/interventions requiring a check or initials to indicate care. As necessary, forms should be supplemented by brief daily notes to avoid appearing unskilled. In some settings allowed weekly entries by regulation, checklists may be used on daily basis. However, if anything unexpected happens, such as issuance of equipment, communication with family, or other unplanned event, a supplemental daily note is written for that day. Authentication is required for all changes in care and supplemental or supporting entries.

APTA Reexamination, Progress Notes/Reports: Periodic entries—weekly, biweekly, or monthly—are compiled based on the daily entries. According to Baetan, Philippi, and Moran (1999), "The focus of the progress report is on the problems identified in the initial evaluation or any new problems that have developed since the last formal reevaluation [*or initial examination/evaluation*]. Documentation describing the skilled intervention provided, complicating factors that may have affected the duration of skilled care, and comparative data."[17]

Significant progress toward functional goals, modification of goals, and completion of goals should be evident. If progress is not demonstrated, justification of this lack of progress as well as justification for continued care with modified goals and plans as indicated must be included. Authentication of any change in care is required.

AUTHOR'S NOTE

Refer to Initial Examination/Evaluation for content categories. For Medicare beneficiaries, recertification for care and payment is based on 30-day (or 60 as applicable) progress reports. However, unless there has been devastating injury or neurological problem (i.e., stroke) most episodes of care should average 30 days. Treatment beyond 30 days may result in higher possibility of review of care by the carrier.

APTA Summation of Episode of Care, Discharge Report/Discharge Evaluation: At the end of the episode of care, patient status, summarized from initial examination/evaluation through the final visit, is required. This summary should address all initial or modified goals and progress or achievement of them. If goals were not achieved, indicate why.

The summation should also include a description of interventions rendered during care, including total number of sessions and the duration (dates) and frequency of the sessions.

The discharge report should also include the patient's discharge disposition, plan for next level of care with recommendations as applicable (including home with home instructions), and any other instructions or training, equipment dispensed, and safety concerns. Authentication is required.

AUTHOR'S NOTE

In entries that include summaries of care without analysis, evaluation, or plans for further care, PTAs may complete the summaries. In circumstances where timely discharge reports are not completed, a summary may be the best way to close out a record. A discharge report or evaluation that includes analysis and plans for further care, requires completion by a PT.

When doing internal utilization review, peer review, or quality assessment, the evaluation and discharge should contain the information necessary to determine if the services were skilled, appropriate, effective, and efficient. If the format is similar, it is easier for the reader to make a determination. In facilities that use outcome assessment measures such as the FIM (Functional Independence Measure) usually used in rehabilitation or FOTO (Focus on Therapeutic Outcomes), usually used in outpatient, values at initial examination and final reexamination should be included. Participation in outcomes systems allows a facility or organization to benchmark their care against other facilities for quality and to easily identify patient progress.

Summary

According to the APTA and AHIMA, medical records should be maintained for all patient/client care, regardless of the payer source, including self pay or pro bono. CMS mandates specific documentation requirements for all Medicare beneficiaries in all venues. The CMS requirements for all settings include the same elements as the APTA Guide to Documentation. All third-party payers require documentation that accurately reflects the PT care rendered and justifies medical necessity, although they may not dictate format or content. The guide categories are Initial Examination and Evaluation/Consultation, Documentation of Continuation of Care, and Documentation of Summation of Episode of Care. The Medicare requirements fit into these categories. Adherence to the APTA and CMS/Medicare guidelines will assist in producing effective documentation that will withstand scrutiny by any reader.

Chapter 4 Review Questions

1. What are the basic requirements for Medicare documentation?

2. Provide ten content elements required in the initial examination and evaluation.

3. Provide five categories of systems review with two examples of content for each.

4. What is the relationship between the patient/client's prior level of function and physical therapy?

5. What are the basic content requirements for a plan of care?

6. From a Medicare perspective, what is recertification and what is the relationship to continuing physical therapy?

7. What does the APTA describe as the Continuation of Care? Provide examples.

8. What is authentication and describe its relationship to documentation?

9. What is the APTA recommended frequency of documentation?

10. What is a problem summary?

Coding and Documentation

Correct coding on the medical/client record is required for all reimbursement. Current Procedural Terminology codes (CPT), developed and owned by the American Medical Association (AMA), are numeric codes for medical procedures. They are required for billing of all medical services including physical therapy. As of fall 2002, the fourth edition of the CPT is in use, and it contains over 10,000 codes. The Healthcare Finance Administration (HCFA, now Center for Medicare and Medicaid, CMS), Common Procedure Coding Systems (HCPCS), Levels I, II, and III, identify specific codes that may be used for billing services delivered to Medicare beneficiaries. Level II codes are not found in the CPT codes. The Level III codes, considered local modifier codes, are scheduled for elimination in the fall of 2003. Also required are International Classification of Disease codes (ICD), which are numeric codes for diseases and pathologies, medical procedures including surgeries, and functionally oriented deficits or conditions. As of fall 2002, ICD-9 (9th revision, Clinical Modifications, 1993, with annual updates in the fall of each calendar year) code versions are in use for physical medicine and physical therapy procedures, although the ICD-10 was published in 2001. The ICD codes were developed by the World Health Organization (WHO) as a way to standardize classification of diseases worldwide (See a sample of ICD-9 codes in Appendix D).

As the CPT codes that describe physical therapy-related procedures have historically been categorized as physical medicine codes, it has been difficult for physical therapists to distinguish themselves from others licensed to administer some of the same procedures. Although recent changes have resulted in several codes unique to physical therapy, it remains incumbent on the physical therapist to prove medical necessity of the service based on consistent matching of CPT codes, ICD-9 codes, and appropriate documentation of what classifies the intervention as skilled.

Another category of code the physical therapist must be familiar with is the Relative Value Resource Based Systems (RVRBS). The RVRBS is a standard system developed by the federal government that assigns a dollar value to medical treatments in order to standardize reimbursement to physicians, with slight adjustments for geographic area. The values are derived from the time and skill (work) required for administration, the related practice cost, and professional liability costs. For several years now, RVRBS values have been established for reimbursement by the federal government for physical therapy (PT) services rendered by Physical Therapists in Private Practice (PTPP, formerly referred to as Physical Therapists in Independent Practice, PTIPs) for outpatients that are Medicare beneficiaries. However, the use of RVRBS is not limited to the Medicare system. RVRBS is used in some states for Medicaid, by managed care organizations (MCOs), and other payers. Medicare calculates the RVRBS payment for PT and other rehabilitation services using the following formula:

EXAMPLE

$$RVU \times GPCI = ARVU$$

where RVU is the relative value unit or component (work, practice, professional liability cost), GPCI is the geographic practice cost indices, and ARVU is the adjusted relative value unit.

Principles of Code Use

One of the challenges of including coding information as a component of documentation is the constant modification of the codes themselves. However, since correct coding is required in order to effect reimbursement, it cannot be ignored. This chapter introduces the concept of coding as it applies to PT. By following the principles and knowing where to obtain the updated information, the physical therapist can ensure that the latest principles and guidelines are consistently applied. Depending on the facility, it may or may not be the PT's responsibility to identify the code numbers. However, in order for a third party such as a billing clerk to correctly code a record, the verbiage must be correct. Based on the size of the CPT and ICD-9 books, learning the verbiage may seem a daunting task. However many facilities use the same categories of patients/clients on a regular basis. Therefore, it is common for facilities to establish a list of frequently used CPT and ICD-9 codes. This list saves time and ensures better consistency throughout facilities. It also eliminates errors if interpretation is left to another party.

Individual Codes

New Codes/Correct Coding Initiatives

It is the PT's responsibility to keep up with the most current coding. Members of the American Physical Therapy Association (APTA) can refer to the APTA web site for updates.

CPT and HCPCS   Make sure the verbiage in the documentation matches the code that will be used in the billing. Always precede specific types of interventions identified colloquially with abbreviations, with the code terminology.

EXAMPLE

Incorrect: CPT 97110: General strengthening, PNF

Correct: CPT 97110: Therapeutic exercise: isotonic strengthening, PNF

ICD-9   The therapist must always include the medical diagnosis established by the physician as the referral diagnosis. However, the PT diagnosis problem for which the therapy is being rendered must be established by the PT since the physician's diagnosis is not always the same as the physical therapist's diagnosis. Regardless, all diagnoses must have verbiage that specifically matches an ICD-9 (or relevant version) code. When appropriate, the PT diagnosis should be functionally oriented and should establish the relevance between the treatment diagnosis, the interventions selected, and the goals established. Do not create "new" diagnoses and always refer to the ICD-9 book for guidance.

EXAMPLE

Same:
  Medical: 812: closed fracture of humerus, upper end
  PT: 812: closed fracture of humerus, upper end
  Referred to PT for treatment of humerus to regain functional use

Different:
  Medical: 812: closed fracture of humerus, upper end
  PT: 781.2 abnormality of gait
  Referred to PT for gait training with quad cane, as can no longer use walker secondary to humerus fracture

ICD-9 Diagnosis Order.   List the code for the primary treatment diagnosis first, followed by the others. Co-morbidities may help justify the need for skilled services.

AUTHOR'S NOTE

The Guide to Physical Therapist Practice *includes medical diagnoses and functional diagnoses commonly used in physical therapy. The ICD-9 code terms are listed in the practice patterns and Appendix D.*

In summer of 2002, new rulings were established by CMS regarding coverage for individuals with 331.0, Alzheimer's and related disorders. It was recognized that individuals with these conditions have the potential to successfully complete and functionally benefit from a course of rehabilitation. However, the patient/client must be able to follow instructions: verbal, gestured, or a combination of the two, and demonstrate functional deficits that can benefit from physical therapy. As PTs do not "treat" Alzheimer's, it remains incumbent on the PT to justify the need for care based on functional deficits and prior level of function as in all patients/clients (i.e., 812 gait abnormality, 728.2 muscular wasting and disuse atrophy).

Matching Codes

ICD-9 and CPT

Once the PT has established the appropriate treatment or PT diagnosis, it should be clear from the verbiage and the code number that they are related. The CMS 1500 form (see Appendix C) allows for services to be specified for each diagnosis.

EXAMPLE

Incorrect:

Medical:	412 old myocardial infarction
PT:	412 old myocardial infarction
Treatment: Gait training:	97116

Correct:

Medical:	412 old myocardial infarction
PT:	781.2 Gait abnormality,
Treatment: Gait training:	97116

Also correct:

Medical:	344.0 quadriplegia
PT:	344.0 quadriplegia
Treatment: Therapeutic exercise:	97110
Neuromuscular reeducation:	97112
Therapeutic activities:	97530

Procedure Specificity

When selecting a code for a procedure, it is important to be as specific as possible. Select the code that best describes the intervention you are using.

EXAMPLE

Incorrect:

Gait training: CPT 97116
Treatment: Balance and posture training

Correct:

Neuromuscular reeducation: CPT 97112
Treatment: Balance and posture training

Time

Most CPTs are defined in 15-minute increments, with each 15-minute segment described as a unit. Depending on the billing form used, the number of units may be required. The total session time should be recorded in the documentation itself.

Medicare B considers each AMA defined CPT code as 8 to 23 minutes, not 15. Therefore, it is recommended that the total time of the treatment session be included in the documentation to accurately represent the time the patient/client actually received treatment. This is also recommended practice for non-Medicare billing purposes as well as liability.

AUTHOR'S NOTE

As a general principle, four or less CPT codes should be billed together. For the majority of procedures, this would represent one hour of treatment. If treatment exceeds one hour or four codes, this must be justified in the documentation. For Medicare Part B, based on the 8- to 23-minute increments, it should be three or less. For timed services that exceed 23 minutes but are less than 38 minutes, two units should be billed. If a specific modality or procedure is less than 8 minutes, indicate this in the notes. However, most interventions are at least 8 minutes in duration.

Modalities and Procedures

Although modalities, such as hot packs or cold packs, are generally not reimbursable alone because application of them is not necessarily considered skilled, they may be when rendered in conjunction with a procedure that is facilitated with their use.

Modifiers

The use of modifiers allows the therapist to indicate when special consideration is needed to demonstrate the need for specific intervention. Modifiers may be used when treatment and evaluation are being performed on the same day or the patient/client has seen a physician and the PT. Some standard modifiers are listed below and can also be found in the DMA CPT manual and Level II Medicare HCPCS manual.

- **GP:** indicates the PT provided the services or care is being delivered under the PT POC
- **GA:** patient/client has been advised in advance that the service is not reasonable and necessary by Medicare standards and it is anticipated that Medicare will deny it
- **GZ:** same as GA but the Medicare beneficiary has been advised in advance
- **GY:** service or procedure is known to be noncovered
- **25:** evaluation and management performed on same day as treatment
- **59:** identifies a distinct service. If the physician has evaluated the patient/client the same day, this would indicate the PT evaluation was separate and distinct.
- **76:** treatment BID

Bundling

Although most procedures and modalities have separate and distinct codes, reimbursement may not be available individually. When a procedure or modality is not paid as distinct and separate, it is considered bundled. Medicare bundles hot packs and cold packs with all other services. CPT code 97602 for nonselective debridement may also be bundled. However, the provider should check with the specific carrier, payer or FI (fiscal intermediary) regarding bundled procedures and codes.

Therapeutic Codes/Procedures

PT Evaluation: 97001. This code is used for PT Evaluation including tests, measures, and analysis and synthesis, to establish a prognosis, plan of care, and appropriate goals based on the findings and anticipated recovery.

PT Reevaluation: 97002. This code is used for PT Reevaluation including tests, measures, and analysis and synthesis, to establish a prognosis, plan of care, and appropriate goals based on the findings and anticipated recovery, when a complete reevaluation is needed, and not in the course of ongoing treatment and regular reassessment for daily recording.

AUTHOR'S NOTE

There is a distinction made between those modalities that require one-on-one administration by the therapist and those that do not. Additionally, the specific body part(s) must be indicated in the documentation for all procedures and modalities. Deficits must be clearly identified, and goals objectively described, with an appropriate treatment plan or plan of care (POC).

Hot Packs/Cold Packs: 97010. For Medicare purposes, this is a bundled code and will not be paid for separately. Justification must be clear in the documentation of the need for the hot pack or cold pack and the expected goal, even if used as an adjunct to another procedure. Specific parameters, including patient position and time must also be included, as well as type and shape of pack. Condition of skin before and after treatment must be noted.

Mechanical Traction: 97012. Used to describe mechanical traction that is set up for the patient and then requires general supervision and adjustment for a period of time. Justification must be clear in the documentation of the need for traction and the expected goal.

Electrical Stimulation: 97014. This code is used for *unattended* electrical stimulation, once the patient/client has been set up. Justification must be clear in the documentation of the need for the stimulation and the expected goal. Specific parameters, including patient position and time must also be included, as well as the type of stimulation, electrode placement, and the machine type. Condition of skin before and after treatment must be noted.

Vasopneumatic Device Therapy: 97016. Used for the administration of Vasopneumatic Compression Device Therapy devices that require parameters to be set prior to use (i.e., mmHg based on blood pressure) and then general supervision over a period of time. Justification must be clear in the documentation of the need for vasopneumatic compression and the expected goal. Specific parameters, including patient position and time must also be included, as well as appropriate measurements of edema using girth and or volumetric measurement. It must be clearly stated when using girth, where the measurements were taken. Treatment must indicate a linear progression of decreasing edema to enable function. Condition of skin before and after treatment must be noted.

Paraffin Bath: 97018. Justification must be clear in the documentation of the need for paraffin bath and the expected goal. Specific parameters, including patient position and time must also be included. Precautions should be clearly indicated and the patient/client appropriately supervised. Condition of skin before and after treatment must be noted.

Microwave Therapy: 97020. Justification must be clear in the documentation of the need for microwave therapy and the expected goal. Specific parameters, including patient position and time must also be included. Precautions should be clearly indicated and the patient/client appropriately supervised. Condition of skin before and after treatment must be noted.

Whirlpool Therapy (non-Hubbard Tanks): 97022. Justification must be clear in the documentation of the need for whirlpool therapy and the expected goal. Specific parameters, including patient position, type of whirlpool used, direction and intensity of jets, water temperature, additives, and time, must also be included. Precautions should be clearly indicated and the patient/client appropriately supervised at all times. Condition of skin before and after treatment must be noted. If being used for wound care, specific conditions and measurements of the wound must be included, with clearly stated goals showing linear progression. If being used to facilitate range of motion (ROM), or reduction in limb volume/edema, justification must be clear.

AUTHOR'S NOTE

As there are new wound care codes, use of them may be warranted. The use of whirlpool for wound care, in the advent of more effective and efficient procedures, is questionable.

Diathermy Treatment: 97024. Justification must be clear in the documentation of the need for diathermy treatment and the expected goal. Specific parameters, including patient position, settings, and time, must also be included as well as appropriate padding to an area and removal of external metals, watches, and the like. Precautions should be clearly indicated and the patient/client appropriately supervised at all times.

Infrared Therapy: 97026. Justification must be clear in the documentation of the need for infrared therapy and the expected goal. Specific parameters, including patient position, settings, and time, must also be included. Precautions should be clearly indicated and the patient/client appropriately supervised.

Ultraviolet Therapy: 97028. Justification must be clear in the documentation of the need for ultraviolet therapy and the expected goal. Specific parameters, including patient position, established dosage based on minimal erythemic dosage, and time must also be included. Precautions should be clearly indicated, such as eye protection, and the patient/client appropriately supervised.

Electrical Stimulation Manual: 97032. Justification must be clear in the documentation of the need for electrical stimulation and the expected goal. Specific parameters including patient position, settings, type of probe or stimulator and time must also be included. Precautions should be clearly indicated and the patient/client appropriately supervised at all times. The skin should be inspected before and after treatment.

Electrical Current Therapy/Iontophoresis: 97033. Justification must be clear in the documentation of the need for electrical current therapy/iontophoresis and the expected goal. Specific parameters, including patient position and time, must also be included as well as the medication used. Precautions should be clearly indicated and the patient/client appropriately supervised at all times. The skin should be inspected before and after.

Contrast Bath Therapy: 97034. Justification must be clear in the documentation of the need for contrast bath therapy and the expected goal. Specific parameters, including patient position, water temperatures, receptacle used, and time in each receptacle and total time, must also be included. Precautions should be clearly indicated and the patient/client appropriately supervised at all times. The skin should be inspected before and after treatment.

Ultrasound Therapy: 97035. Justification must be clear in the documentation of the need for ultrasound therapy and the expected goal. Specific parameters, including patient position, area treated, type of ultrasound (i.e., pulsed vs. continuous), transmission medium, intensity, and time, must also be included. Precautions should be clearly indicated and the patient/client appropriately supervised at all times.

Hydrotherapy/Hubbard Tank: 97036. Justification must be clear in the documentation of the need for Hubbard Tank Hydrotherapy and the expected goal. Specific parameters, including patient position, water temperature, intensity, and direction of jets, water additives, and time, must also be included. Precautions should be clearly indicated and the patient/client appropriately supervised at all times.

Physical Therapy Treatment: 97039. This is a nonspecific code and, therefore, should be avoided. It should be used only if a procedure is being used that does not fall into any other category.

Manual Therapy: 97140. This code includes manual therapy/mobilization/manipulation, manual lymphatic drainage, and manual traction to one or more regions. Justification must be clear in the documentation of the need for the specific procedure and the expected goal. Specific parameters, including patient position, methodology, and post-therapy procedures such as compression wrapping must also be included. Precautions should be clearly indicated with the patient constantly attended as manual therapy is hands-on throughout. The coding is by 15-minute increments regardless of number of areas treated.

Therapeutic Exercise: 97110. All categories of skilled therapeutic exercise are covered by this code to one or more areas. It covers strengthening (not general in nature) and exercises to develop endurance and flexibility. It is imperative that the documentation and POC include the term therapeutic exercise before listing the specific types employed with the patient/client. For justification of the need for skilled exercise, specific exercise parameters, applicable hand placement, technique name, and patient/client must be included. The exercises must be appropriate for the level of strength/muscle performance the patient/client demonstrates, and linked ultimately to function. Strength should be expressed in fractions, which are more universally understood by nonprofessionals than verbiage. One of the most common scales expresses strength in a range from 0/5 to 5/5, with 5/5 being the strongest, and 0/5 representing no muscle contraction. Avoid using goals for strength that state "increase strength by 1/2 grade." Instead, link the strength to function and state the expectation.

EXAMPLE

Increase strength from 3/5 to 4/5 in LEs to enable stair climbing into home.

Range of motion (ROM) should also be expressed in numbers. Goniometric measurements, using the appropriate goniometer, are the most reliable compared to visual estimates. ROM is best stated in fractions, with the available ROM, active (AROM) or passive (PROM), listed over the total "normal" ROM. If the full AROM should be 180° and the patient/client demonstrates 90°, it should be recorded as 90°/180°. Avoid using terms such as "increase by 10%." Instead, as in strength, list the numbers and link to function.

EXAMPLE

Increase ROM from 90°/180° degrees to 160°/180° in order to . . .

Neuromuscular Reeducation: 97112. Justification must be clear in the documentation of the need for neuromuscular reeducation. The code is used for reeducation of balance, coordination, kinesthetic sense, posture, and proprioception for activities performed in sitting and standing.

Aquatic Therapy/Exercises: 97113. This code is intended for individual patient/client sessions that are in water. For justification of the need for skilled aquatics, specific exercise parameters and why the patient/client requires a water-based environment must be included.

Gait Training: 97116. Justification must be clear in the documentation for the need for gait training. Although many carriers and fiscal intermediaries allow the term ambulation to be used to describe "skilled walking assessment and intervention," the CPT code term is gait. For consistency, therefore, and indication that the activity is the same, the use of the term "gait" for assessment and training purposes is recommended. The term "walking" is never considered skilled and should be avoided unless the patient/client is being quoted. "Skilling" gait requires the assessment and training of all gait characteristics with appropriate goals including: base of support (BOS); arm swing; swing phase; initial contact; stance; deviations; level of the pelvis; weight bearing and acceptance of weight on the limb; stride length; cadence; posture; assistive devices; balance; surfaces; safety; ability to change directions and negotiate or avoid obstacles; opening and closing doors; asymmetry; distance; sequencing; leg length discrepancies; extent of total effort patient/client is exerting if assistance is needed; and speed. Normal gait speed = 82 m/min.

Massage Therapy/Therapeutic Massage: 97124. Massage should be referred to as therapeutic massage in the documentation. The body part/area should be clearly stated as well as the relationship between the therapeutic and the expected outcome. It is usually used adjunctively to decrease spasm, increase joint range, decrease edema, and restore muscle function. Types of strokes should also be included in the documentation. With appropriate justification, this code may be used for postural drainage techniques if it is necessary for it to be done by PT.

Group Therapeutic Procedures: 97150. Used when patients/clients are receiving skilled services in a group (2 or more) with others requiring similar services (same plan of care). The PT must indicate in the documentation the specific treatment, how it will result in stated goals for the specific patient, and the size of the group.

AUTHOR'S NOTE

As of spring 2002, CMS/Medicare reviewed the group therapy code. They issued a transmittal indicating that even if all patients/clients are not receiving the same treatment, this code should be used if the PT is attending to multiple patients/clients in the same time period. Therapist must be in constant attendance, but not involved in one-on-one physical contact. However, according to the APTA, part of the session may be billed individually for direct one-on-one intervention. (Transmittal: CMS 1753 CR 2126)

Therapeutic Activities, Direct: 97530. This category covers direct functional activities, such as lifting, carrying, reaching, catching, overhead activities, and bending, employed when a patient/client demonstrates limitations in strength, flexibility, range of motion, balance, and/or coordination. The documentation must show the relationship between the activities and the stated goals.

Transfer training or transitional movements may also be included in this category. Each type of transfer necessary for function should be included (i.e., sit to and from stand, stand and pivot, partial stand and pivot, sliding board use, standing disks, mechanical lifts, sit to and from supine, supine to and from long sit). The degree of patient/client ability must be stated clearly and reflected in the goals. Colloquially for physical therapy, patient/client ability has been stated in terms of assistance needed, which translates into patient/client ability. The terms are: independent (I), supervisor(s), minimally dependent or minimal assistance, moderately dependent or moderate assistance, maximally dependent or maximal assistance, and total dependence or total assistance. Medicare recommends the use of the terms limited and extensive, with limited corresponding to minimal and extensive corresponding to all other more dependent terms. However, percentage (%) of patient effort is required for all descriptions. Percentage should always be expressed in the evaluation to establish a baseline, with goals indicating decreasing percentage in a linear fashion. This covers dynamic activities and assumes one-on-one constant attendance. Essential functional activities—those activities that a patient/client needs to do rather than wants to do— are applicable in this category.

Sensory Integration: 97533. Justification must be clear in the documentation of the need for sensory integration. The code is used for enhancement of sensory processing, promoting appropriate responses between the patient/client and the environment. This activity requires constant attendance with one-on-one care, in 15-minute increments.

Selective Debridement: 97601. This code includes removal of devitalized tissue from wound or selective debridement without anesthesia (i.e., high pressure water jet, sharp debridement). Justification must be clear in the documentation of the need for selective debridement based on the description of the wound and devitalized tissue.

Non-Selective Debridement: 97602. This code includes general, nonspecific removal of tissue. For Medicare purposes, this is a bundled code.

Wheelchair Management Training/Propulsion: 97542. This code is used for skilled instruction and adaptation determination of both temporary or permanent confinement to a manual or power wheelchair or power-operated vehicle (scooter). When documenting for manual chairs, all appropriate aspects must be included, such as ability to transfer in and out of (including falls, bed, toilet, other chairs, other surfaces, ramps, cars/buses/trains), manipulation of any of the parts (brakes or power controls), terrain (even/uneven, indoor/outdoor), door opening and closing, all directions including turns, and folding/unfolding. The training of caretakers in all aspects of wheelchair use may also be applicable to this code. The same parameters are applied for power mobility appropriate for the types of controls and adaptations. Essential functional activities—those activities that a patient/client needs to do rather than wants to do—are also applicable to this category.

Cognitive Skills Development: 97532. Justification must be clear in the documentation of the need for cognitive skills development, such as improved memory, reasoning, problem solving, and attention to tasks. This activity requires constant attendance with one-on-one care, billed in 15-minute increments.

Orthotic Training: 97504. Justification must be clear in the documentation of the need for orthotic training and fitting and the expected goal. The type of orthotic and body area must be included (i.e., upper extremity [UE], lower extremity [LE], and trunk) and billed in 15-minute increments. Precautions should be clearly indicated and the patient/client appropriately supervised.

AUTHOR'S NOTE

A durable medical equipment (DME) number may be needed in order to bill for the actual orthosis. Treatment under this code may not be reimbursable for multiple sessions.

According to the First Coast Medicare Web site: Orthotic training (CPT code 97504) for a lower extremity performed during the same visit as gait training (CPT code 97116) or self-care/home management training (CPT code 97535) should not be reported unless documentation in the medical record shows that distinct treatments were rendered. In addition, the casting and strapping codes should not be reported in addition to code 97504. If casting and strapping of a fracture, injury, or dislocation is performed, procedure codes 29000–29590 should be reported. Please refer to the LMRP policy (29580) for further guidelines regarding strapping.

Prosthetic Training: 97520. Justification must be clear in the documentation of the need for prosthetic training and the expected goal. The type of prosthetic and body area must be included (i.e., upper extremity [UE] or lower extremity [LE]) and billed in 15-minute increments. Precautions should be clearly indicated and the patient/client appropriately supervised. The pattern of use must be clearly indicated and any gait deviations, pressure concerns, and functional challenges for the LE listed. For the UE, pattern of use, pressure concerns, and functional challenges must be included.

Self Care/Home Management Training: 97542. Justification must be clear in the documentation of the need for self-care/home management training. This includes activities such as activities of daily living (ADL), meal preparation, use of assistive or adaptive devices and technologies, and safety. Precautions should be clearly indicated and the patient/client appropriately supervised. Billing should be listed in 15-minute increments.

Community/Work Reintegration: 97537. Justification must be clear in the documentation of the need for community/work reintegration. Reintegration includes developing incremental activities of daily living (IADL) skills, such as shopping, negotiating transportation, managing monetary transactions, vocational and avocational activities, work environment and ergonomic considerations, and work task analysis. Precautions should be clearly indicated. This activity requires constant attendance with one-on-one care and should be billed in 15-minute increments. Medicare may not reimburse for all activities covered by this code based on the concept of essential function.

Work Hardening: 97545. Justification must be clear in the documentation of the need for work hardening and the expected goal. Specific parameters, activities, and time must also be included. Precautions should be clearly indicated and the patient/client appropriately supervised. This code is used for the initial two hours of work hardening. Medicare does not reimburse for work hardening.

Work Hardening Add-on: 97546. This code would be used for time beyond the initial two hours, and is billed in 1-hour increments.

Prosthetic Check-out: 97703. Prosthetic check-out covers check out for an established patient for a prosthesis or orthosis and should be billed in 15-minute increments.

Physical Performance Test: 97750. Physical performance test covers performance tests, such as functional capacity assessments and other performance measures with written report (i.e., isokinetic testing).

Unlisted Physical Medicine/Rehabilitation Service or Procedure: 97799. This code would be used for an unlisted service.

Apply Neurostimulator: 64550. Application of a neurostimulator may include a bone stimulator or functional electrical stimulation, but not TENS unit.

Biofeedback Training/Any method: 90901. Biofeedback training/any method covers external methods. Justification and need must be clear in the documentation. Specific patient positioning, parameters, electrode or feedback device placement, time, and goals must be included.

Biofeedback Training Peri/Uro/Rect: 90911. Biofeedback training peri/uro/rect covers specific training for the perineals, urethral sphincter, or anorectal sphincter, with specialized equipment. Specific patient positioning, parameters, electrode or feedback device placement, time, and goals must be included. Medicare may cover this for incontinence with appropriate documentation and justification.

Limb Muscle Testing, Manual: (95831); Hand Muscle Testing, Manual: (95832); Body Muscle Testing, Manual: (95833–834). Codes 95831–95834 are self-explanatory. It is the PTs responsibility to get clarification from the payer regarding the use of these versus the PT evaluation code. In cases such as peripheral nerve injury in a limb, post-operative hand management or spinal cord injury, these codes may be preferable to the evaluation code.

Range of Motion Measurements: 95851–852. It is the PTs responsibility to get clarification from the payer regarding the use of these versus the PT evaluation code. In cases such as multiple trauma in which multiple ranges must be obtained, these codes may be preferable to the PT evaluation code.

Motion Analysis, Video 3d: 96000. Justification must be clear in the documentation of the need for motion analysis, video 3d and the outcomes from the assessment as well as goals.

Motion Test with Foot Pressure Measurement: 96001. Justification must be clear of the need for motion analysis of dynamic foot pressure measurement during gait. The goals and outcomes from the assessment should also be included.

Dynamic Surface EMG: 96002. Justification must be clear in the documentation of the need for dynamic surface EMG during walking and other functional activities. The goals and outcomes from the assessment should also be included. This is calculated in increments up to 12 minutes.

Dynamic Fine Wire EMG: 96003. Justification must be clear in the documentation of the need for dynamic fine wire EMG during walking and other functional activities for 1 muscle. The goals and outcomes from the assessment should also be included.

Developmental Test, Limb: 96110; Developmental Test, Extremity: 96111; Neurobehavior Status Exam: 96115. Generally, codes 96110, 96111, and 96115, are covered under the PT evaluation code. With appropriate certification, based on state licensing, PTs with special certification may perform and receive reimbursement for EMG/NCV under codes 95860–95937 from Medicare.

AUTHOR'S NOTE

Before using any code to bill for procedures, check with the carrier/FI to determine if the service is covered. Identification of a procedure by code does not automatically qualify it for payment.

Non-Covered Conditions and Services as listed on CMS Web site

It is the responsibility of the therapist to be aware of medical conditions and services not covered by the third party payer. Regardless of the documentation, noncovered services will not be paid regardless of therapist efforts or goals. Examples **of non-covered** services and conditions in the **Medicare Program** include:

1) Vertebral Axial Decompression (VAD) therapy is considered "investigational" and is a noncovered service under Florida Medicare.

2) General exercises to promote overall fitness and flexibility and activities to provide diversion or general motivation.

3) Work hardening/conditioning **(CPT codes 97545-97546)**

4) Electrotherapy performed for the treatment of facial nerve paralysis in the application of electrical stimulation **(97014)**.

5) Electrotherapy for the treatment of facial nerve paralysis, commonly known as Bell's Palsy **(ICD-9 code 351.0)**

6) Diathermy **(97024)** or ultrasound **(97035)** heat treatments performed for respiratory conditions or diseases **(ICD-9 codes 460-519.9)** are investigational under the Medicare program.

7) General exercise programs to improve a patient's general cardiovascular fitness; pulmonary rehabilitation; cardiac rehabilitation; or a maintenance program of therapeutic activities.

8) Aquatic therapy with therapeutic exercise **(97113)** should not be billed when there is not one-on-one contact between therapist and patient.

9) Diapulse and Rolfing **(97799)** treatment is noncovered.

10) Noncovered ICD-9 codes, i.e., Bell's Palsy

11) Hot packs or cold packs unless bundled and an integral component of other intervention

Coding Guidelines

Providers may report Evaluation and Management services on the same day as physical medicine treatments provided the services are separately identifiable.

AUTHOR'S NOTE

If billed with modifier codes.

There is a clear relationship between CPT coding, ICD-9 (or appropriate ICD edition coding), and documentation. In order to receive reimbursement, the ICD code must be related to the treatment rendered. The treatment rendered must be described in verbiage that matches the CPT codes in order to appropriately code the billing. However, regardless of the accuracy of the CPT and ICD coding, the documentation must also support the medical necessity of the skilled PT intervention in an appropriate time frame. Unless there is devastating illness or injury, or the patient/client is in a pre-approved program of prescribed time, most care should be planned for episodes of 30 days or less.

Understanding the basic concepts of coding and application of them, will not guarantee reimbursement. It is up to the therapist to justify all care by entering into the record that skilled services were required, goals were reasonable and reached (preferably in a linear manner), care was reasonable and necessary, and the therapy was both effective and efficient.

Summary

The Correct Coding Initiative of 1998 (CCI) required the use of CPT codes for all Medicare billing of rehabilitation services, as do all payers. HCFA, now CMS, developed the HCPCS codes for those codes not included in the AMA CPT coding. In order to ensure reimbursement, the correct procedural codes must be used for all physical therapy services, many of which are general physical medicine codes.

The correct combination of CPT codes, ICD-9 diagnostic codes, CPT matching verbiage describing the procedures rendered in the documentation, emphasis on function, ongoing justification of the medical necessity for skilled PT, and matched billing dates, will assist the PT in ensuring reimbursement based on the documentation.

In those instances in which the PT is not performing the CPT coding or billing, it is critical that the individual(s) handling the billing understand correct coding. If the PT is familiar enough with the codes and appropriate terminology to use them appropriately, an "outsider" can more easily do the coding. Electronic or computerized systems can be designed to facilitate automatic coding, as inclusion of codes with correction description on pre-printed forms.

Chapter 5 Review Questions

1. What is a CPT code? Explain the application in physical therapy.

2. What is an ICD-9 code? Explain the application in physical therapy.

3. What is the relationship between the CPT codes and ICD-9 codes?

4. What is the medical diagnosis?

5. What is the physical therapy diagnosis or physical therapy problem?

6. What is the relationship between the medical diagnosis and the physical therapy diagnosis (problem)?

7. What is a code modifier? Explain the role of modifiers in the billing process.

8. What are the time increments for CPT code procedures for Medicare billing versus non-Medicare billing?

9. Relative to CPT codes, explain the difference between attended and unattended procedures.

10. What are the risks of billing for noncovered procedures?

Standardized Forms and Content

The use of standardized forms for documentation and billing purposes aids in maintaining consistency within an organization or facility, as well as between therapy personnel. Blank forms or pages lead to inconsistency and omission of information that may be crucial in supporting medical necessity for skilled physical therapy (PT) services. Although pre-made forms (or formats in the electronic medical record) do not guarantee the quality of content, if keys or legends are provided in each category, the information is more likely to be included. The APTA's *Guide to Documentation* includes sample forms (see Appendix E). The forms in the guide are not detailed (with exception of the history) and therefore should be used only as a guide to develop forms that best suit the facility's needs. This is applicable to manual entry forms as well as electronically generated forms or formats.

There are a variety of forms required or strongly recommended for billing of services depending on the payer. Examples include Medicare's 700 series forms (see Appendix B), the CMS 1450 (UB 92), and the CMS 1500 form (see Appendix C). The forms come with the instructions pre-printed on them. Adherence to the instructions will help to ensure that they are completed appropriately. The 700 series forms are used in skilled nursing facilities (SNFs), certified rehabilitation facilities (CORFs), and rehabilitation agencies (RAs). The CMS 1500 form is used for all other outpatient or Part B services rendered in other settings. The 700 series forms are available and were developed by CMS over a decade ago in an attempt to standardize billing and documentation. They are not required, rather the information requested on the 700 series forms is required. The authors of this text recommend that the forms be used with minor adaptations. If a facility decides that the form is too limiting because of space, the new form that is designed should resemble the original form as much as possible. All the information required on the series forms should be on the self-designed form and it is recommended that the PT contact the fiscal intermediary (FI) to get approval for use of a self-designed form. Regardless of the form used, the goal of the provider should be to submit a clean—error free—claim. If information is requested to support the bill, it should be self-explanatory and reinforce the information and charges on the claim form.

In addition to the use of forms, the terminology used in the documentation must be universally understood by all possible record "readers," yet sophisticated enough to justify the skilled care rendered. In this context, there are terms that can and should be used and terms that should be avoided. Terms that may be used by the therapist in conversation, should not necessarily appear in the documentation. According to Baetan, Philippi, and Moran (1999) "Functional phrase alternatives are terms or phrases that convey to the reviewer the skilled nature of the service provided. . . . the concept of using functional phrase alternatives can be expanded to all practice setting."[18]

Appropriate identification of patient/client problems with relevant goals is another key to successful documentation. Although goals should be functionally oriented, impairment-based goals should be included as they relate to function. The goals of the patient/client or caregiver(s) need to be addressed in the documentation. However, they must be achievable and appropriate for the episode of care. The therapist should provide goals for the episode in which they are providing care only. If a continuum is expected (i.e., acute care to inpatient rehabilitation to home health to outpatient), each therapist establishes the goals for the setting and time period for which the patient/client is under their care. In the discharge or summation of care, the therapist should address the need for the patient/client to receive continuing services in the next setting.

Categories and Appropriate Terminology

What to Avoid

Avoid using the terms "walking" when referring to gait training and "maintain" (unless used in the context of balance ability). Also avoid repeated statements that patient is not progressing, noncompliant, or uncooperative, unless the intention is to discontinue the PT.

Avoid using nondescriptive terms such as patient is "the same," "not improving," or "still not compliant."

Avoid terms without clear meaning, such as "uncooperative, confused, agitated, noncompliant," unless the plan is to discharge (DC). Other terms without clear meaning include tolerated well; general increase in; general improvement, strengthening, or supervision; poor carry through; declined in function; not responding to treatment; improved (unless objective data follows); and increased or decreased pain without reference to a scale that can be measured and relationship to function.

What to Include

Descriptive, Objective Terminology and Data/Measures　Examples of descriptive, objective terminology and data/measures include functionally oriented goals; distances, deficits with progress toward goals, based on the Disablement Model, and functional limitations and disabilities that can be impacted during the episode of care by resolving impairments.

For Medicare purposes, focus on essential function versus nonessential function, especially in inpatient and home health. Once patient/client has progressed to outpatient (OP), community safety must also be addressed. Use comparisons that illustrate progress and provide instruction in precautions, independent exercise, and caregiver training. Use skilled terminology that matches CPT codes for interventions (i.e., therapeutic exercise, gait training). Terminology as indicated in the *Guide to Physical Therapist Practice* is also acceptable and should include application of practice patterns for goals, interventions, and progress.

Range of motion (ROM) should be expressed as fractions, indicating total "normal" range based on a standard, i.e., 120°/180°, 45°/90°, and so on. ROM goals should be written to indicate the goal ROM and the reason it is necessary.

EXAMPLE

Increase AROM L shoulder flexion from 95°/180° to 180°/180° in order to return to job as house painter.

Strength should be expressed in fractions based on a standardized scale such as the 0/5 to 5/5 scale. Strength goals should be written to indicate the goal strength and the reason it is necessary.

EXAMPLE

Increase strength of L shoulder flexion from 3/5 to 5/5 in order to return to job as house painter, and sustain full flexion of the shoulder up to 6 hours/day.

Records should also include numeric expression of assistance with component for which help is needed (i.e., minimal or limited assistance of 25%, moderate or extensive assistance of 50%, maximal or extensive assistance of 75%, or total assistance 100%), applied for transfers, transitional movements, gait, wheelchair mobility, balance, or other objective measures of gait with use of consistent terminology. Since the CPT code is gait training, consistently use gait throughout the entry, avoiding introduction of the term ambulation. Walking is not a skilled term.

Please refer to Chapters 4 and 5 for additional information on content. The initial examination is presented again as an overview, because its importance cannot be stressed enough. If the appropriate content is in the initial examination/evaluation, including objective measures, identified physical therapy problems, clear delineation of the patient's deficits that can be impacted in a reasonable amount of time (frequency and duration), with appropriate goals and interventions, the appropriate baseline will be established for the total episode of care.

Initial Examination

Clarification of history that is relevant includes co-morbidities and medications that may affect the patient and their specific relationship to PT. The identified deficits or status are listed below by category.

Problems.   Problems include impairments, functional limitations, disabilities, or a general summary of problems based on findings from tests and measures resulting from interpretation of the data.

Goals/Functional Outcomes/Prognosis.   What the patient/client will achieve as a result of the intervention and the potential for achievement.

Interventions (Plan).   What the therapist will do with the patient/client based on terminology used in CPT coding preceding any other descriptors that may not be universally understood.

Timelines and Anticipated Dates/Duration.   Total length of time it is anticipated to take to achieve outcomes, or duration based on pre-authorization or pre-determination. Based on progress and patient/client need, the therapist can always appeal to the provider for additional sessions. Indicate dates versus number of days or weeks, although either may be acceptable.

Frequency of Visits to Achieve Goals.   Visits or sessions per day, per week, or as appropriate. Prognosis or rehabilitation potential that is relative only to the PT. It should always be at least "good" if the PT is establishing the goals. If PT establishes that it is "fair" based on severity of medical condition, status should be clear in the initial examination information.

Guidelines for Content and Forms as Listed in CMS Carrier Manual (cms.gov)

AUTHOR'S NOTE

Although this information is Medicare specific, it is applicable in most settings for all payers and patients/clients. It includes clear examples and explanations of guidelines for skilled PT services.

Providers of Medicare Outpatient Services

Hospitals, rural primary care hospitals, skilled nursing facilities, home health agencies, hospice programs, or certified outpatient rehabilitation facilities (CORF), clinic, rehabilitation agency, physical therapists in private practice.

Coverage for Outpatient Services

Services are covered only if they are reasonable and necessary for the diagnosis or treatment of illness or injury or to improve the function of a malformed body member. Thus, there must be potential for restoration or improvement of lost or impaired functions.

Examples of Noncovered Services   Services involving repetitive services that do not require the skilled services of nurses or therapists, e.g., maintenance programs, general conditioning, or ambulation, are not covered. These services could be performed in the patient's residence by non-medical personnel such as family members. It is not reasonable and necessary for such services to be performed in an ambulatory care setting by CORF personnel.

Medicare and As Applicable State to State by Payer for Non-Medicare

Referral for Treatment

To become a patient of an outpatient facility, the beneficiary must be under the care of a physician who certifies that the beneficiary needs skilled rehabilitation services. The referring physician must advise PT of the beneficiary's medical history, current diagnosis and medical findings, desired rehabilitation goals (may be established by the PT in conjunction with), and any contraindications to specific activity or intensity of rehabilitation services.

Plan of Treatment

PT services must be furnished under a written plan of care (See Chapter 4).

Certification and Recertification Including Plan of Treatment (Plan of Care)

Treatment established by a physician. The physician may be either a physician associated with the facility (as in a CORF) or the referring physician if he/she provides a detailed plan of treatment (designed in conjunction with the physical therapist) that meets the following requirements:

1. The plan of treatment must contain the diagnosis (referring medical diagnosis and the established PT diagnosis or PT problem established by the PT and preferably functionally oriented) type (interventions stated in CPT or HCPCS verbiage), amount (parameters), frequency (× per day, week, etc.), and duration of services (total length of time for episode of care or length of stay [LOS]) to be performed and the anticipated rehabilitation goals, emphasizing function that can be achieved in a reasonable time (preferably 30 days or less, unless acute co-morbidities or devastating condition such as acute CVA or multiple trauma).

2. Indicate services are or were required because the patient needed skilled rehabilitation services (for an acute condition or recent exacerbation resulting in functional decline from a chronic condition, or an improvement in condition or cognition allowing participation in PT not previously possible).

3. Be sufficiently detailed to permit an independent evaluation of the patient's specific need for the indicated skilled PT services and of the likelihood that he/she will derive meaningful benefit from them (goals must be significant from a functional perspective).

4. Indicate the services are or were reasonable and necessary to the treatment of the patient's condition and not harmful (identifying all precautions and any contraindications).

5. Be reviewed by the physician at least once every 30 days or initial 60 days for a CORF. Following the review, the physician must certify that the plan of treatment is being followed and that the patient is making progress in attaining the established rehabilitation goals (established by the PT in conjunction with the physician). When the patient has reached a point where no further progress is being made toward one or more of the goals, Medicare coverage ends for that aspect of the plan of treatment.

6. Since the certification is closely associated with the plan of treatment, the same physician who establishes or reviews the plan must certify the necessity for the services. Obtain the certification at the time the plan of treatment is established or as soon thereafter as possible.

7. Obtain the recertification at the time the plan of treatment is reviewed since the same interval (at least once every 30 or 60 days depending on outpatient setting) is required for the review of the plan. Recertifications are signed by the physician who reviews the plan of treatment and has examined the patient/client in the recertification period. The PT may choose the form and manner of obtaining timely recertification, i.e., electronic, mail, and fax.

AUTHOR'S NOTE

Sending recertifications out a few days prior to the due date with a note of explanation and a return addressed enveloped with an arrow "sticky" indicating where the signature goes, or faxing and then sending it out to be signed, may prevent undue delay.

Any changes to this plan must be made in writing and must be signed by the physician and therapist. Changes to the plan may also be made pursuant to oral orders given by the attending physician to a qualified physical therapist.

Changes to such plans also may be made pursuant to oral orders by the physical therapist to another qualified physical therapist, or by the therapist to a registered professional nurse on your staff. Such changes must be immediately recorded in the patient's record and must be signed by the individual receiving the orders. While the physician may change a plan of treatment established by the therapist providing such services, the therapist may or may not alter a plan of treatment established by a physician.

AUTHOR'S NOTE

The patient's plan normally need not be forwarded with the claim, but is retained in the provider's file. The provider must certify on the billing form that the plan is on file. The plan and other documentation must be submitted upon request.

Make sure the plan is established or reduced to writing either by the person who established the plan or by you when you make a written record of that person's oral orders, before treatment begins. The plan must be promptly signed by the ordering physician, and therapist, or speech pathologist and incorporated into the patient's clinical record.

Method and Disposition of Certifications and Delayed Certification

For information on method and disposition of certifications and delayed certification please refer to Chapter 4.

Medicare

271.1. Physical Therapy Services: Conditions of Coverage

To be covered, physical therapy services must relate directly and specifically to the plan of treatment described in §270.3, and be reasonable and necessary to the treatment of the individual's illness or injury. Services related to activities for the general well being and welfare of patients (i.e., general exercises to promote overall fitness and flexibility and activities to provide diversion or general motivation) do not constitute physical therapy services for Medicare purposes.

According to the Guide to Physical Therapist Practice *there are 5 elements of patient care: Examination, Evaluation, Diagnosis, Prognosis, and Intervention.*

Evaluation   The evaluation is an integral component of physical therapy services. It is the clinical judgments of the PT based on the synthesis of data/information/findings to establish the diagnosis, prognosis, and plan of care. It establishes the baseline data (including identified functional problems and related impairments that can be impacted by skilled PT intervention) necessary for assessing expected rehabilitation potential, setting realistic (functionally oriented) goals, and measuring progress. The evaluation of the patient's condition must form the basis for the physical therapy treatment goals. A physical therapy initial evaluation (excluding routine screening) is covered when it is reasonable and necessary for the qualified physical therapist to determine if there is an expectation that either restorative or maintenance services are appropriate for the patient's condition. When a patient exhibits a demonstrable change in physical functional ability, reevaluations are covered to reestablish appropriate treatment goals (Reevaluations are also covered for ongoing assessment of the patient's rehabilitation needs). Initial evaluations or reevaluations that are determined reasonable and necessary are covered even though the expectations are not realized or when the evaluation determines that skilled rehabilitation is not needed.

Evaluations only, without justification for intervention may not be reimbursed.

Reasonable and Necessary   In order for services to be considered reasonable and necessary, the services must be considered under accepted standards of medical practice to be a specific and effective treatment for the patient's condition.

The services must be of such a level of complexity and sophistication or the condition of the patient must be such that the services required can be safely and effectively performed only by or under the supervision of a qualified physical therapist. Services that do not require the performance or supervision of a physical therapist are not considered reasonable or necessary physical therapy services even if they are performed or supervised by a physical therapist.

There must be an expectation that the condition will improve significantly in a reasonable (and generally predictable) period of time based on the assessment made by the physician of the patient's restoration potential after any needed consultation with the qualified physical therapist. Alternatively, the services must be necessary to establish a safe and effective maintenance program required in connection with a specific disease state. The amount, frequency, and duration of the services must be reasonable.

When the intermediary determines the services furnished were of a type that could have been safely or effectively performed only by or under the supervision of a qualified physical therapist, it presumes that such services were properly supervised. However, this assumption may be rebutted. If, in the course of processing claims, the intermediary finds that physical therapy services are not being furnished under proper supervision, the intermediary denies the claim and brings this matter to the attention of the Division of Health Standards and Quality of the CMS RO.

Medicare will not reimburse for PT student-rendered care. However, the student may assist the PT if the PT is directly supervising and not engaged in treating other patients at the same time.

Claims for physical therapy services denied because the services are not considered reasonable and necessary are excluded from coverage and are thus subject to consideration under the waiver of liability provision in §1879 of the Act.

Types of Therapy

Restorative Therapy To constitute physical therapy, a service must be reasonable and necessary to the treatment of the individual's illness. If an individual's expected restoration potential is insignificant in relation to the extent and duration of physical therapy services required to achieve such potential, the services are not considered reasonable and necessary. In addition, there must be an expectation that the patient's condition will improve significantly in a reasonable (and generally predictable) period of time. If at any point in the treatment of an illness it is determined that the expectations will not materialize, the services are no longer considered reasonable and necessary and are excluded from coverage.

Maintenance Program The repetitive services required to maintain function generally do not involve complex and sophisticated physical therapy procedures and do not require the judgment and skill of a qualified physical therapist for safety and effectiveness. However, in certain instances, the specialized knowledge and judgment of a qualified physical therapist may be required to establish a maintenance program. For example, a Parkinson's disease patient who has not been under a restorative physical therapy program may require the services of a physical therapist to determine the most effective type of exercise to maintain the patient's present functional level.

In such situations, the following services constitute physical therapy:

- The initial evaluation of the patient's needs;
- The design by the qualified physical therapist of a maintenance program appropriate to the capacity and tolerance of the patient and the treatment objectives of the physician;
- The instruction of the patient or supportive personnel, i.e., aides, nursing personnel or family members, if furnished on an outpatient basis, in carrying out the program; and reevaluations as required.

If a patient has been under a restorative physical therapy program, the physical therapist regularly reevaluates the condition and adjusts the exercise program. The physical therapist should have already designed the required maintenance program and instructed the patient, supportive personnel, or family members, if the services have been furnished on an outpatient basis, in implementing the program before it is determined that no further restoration is possible. Therefore, when the therapist does not establish a maintenance program until after the restorative physical therapy program has been completed, no further physical therapy services are reasonable and necessary. Therefore, establishing such a program is not reasonable and necessary to the treatment of the patient's condition and is not covered.

271.2 Application of Guidelines (From CMS Medicare Carriers Manual)

Coding should generally apply to "more common modalities in which the reasonableness and necessity of physical therapy services is a significant issue."

Medicare Considerations

Hot Pack, Hydrocollator, Infra-Red Treatments, Paraffin Baths, and Whirlpool Baths Heat treatments of this type and whirlpool baths do not ordinarily require the skills of a qualified physical therapist. However, in a particular case, the skills, knowledge, and judgment of a qualified physical therapist might be required in such treatments or baths, e.g., when the patient's condition is complicated by circulatory deficiency, areas of desensitization, open wounds, or other complications. Also, if such treatments are given prior to but as an integral part of a skilled physical therapy procedure, they are part of the physical therapy service.

AUTHOR'S NOTE

However, hot pack treatments and other modalities may be bundled for payment (see Chapter 5) and not be individually reimbursed.

Gait Training   Gait evaluation and training furnished to a patient whose ability to walk has been impaired by neurological, muscular, or skeletal abnormality requires the skills of a qualified physical therapist. However, if gait evaluation and training cannot reasonably be expected to significantly improve the patient's ability to walk, such services are not considered reasonable and necessary. Repetitious exercises to improve gait or maintain strength and endurance and assisted walking are appropriately provided by supportive personnel (i.e., aides or nursing personnel) and do not require the skills of a qualified physical therapist.

It is necessary to include skilled terminology when evaluating gait, describing dependence versus independence, all gait deviations, and need for assistive devices or adaptive equipment.

Ultrasound, Shortwave Diathermy (SWD), and Microwave Diathermy (MWD) Treatments   These modalities must always be performed by or under the supervision of a qualified physical therapist. Therefore, such treatments constitute physical therapy.

AUTHOR'S NOTE

Ultrasound requires constant attendance from a coding perspective, but SWD and MWD do not.

Range of Motion Tests   Only the qualified physical therapist may perform range of motion tests, and such tests constitute physical therapy.

AUTHOR'S NOTE

Objective measurements must be provided indicating available active or passive ROM measured over normal ranges for the joint. They should be stated in fractions, and ultimately relate to lack of function as the reason for care.

Therapeutic Exercises   Therapeutic exercises that must be performed by or under the supervision of the qualified physical therapist because of either the type of exercise employed or the condition of the patient constitute physical therapy.

Range of motion exercises require the skills of a qualified physical therapist only if:

1. They are part of the active treatment of a specific disease which has resulted in a loss or restriction of mobility (as evidenced by physical therapy notes showing the degree of motion lost and the degree to be restored) and;

2. Such exercises, either because of their nature or the condition of the patient, may only be performed safely and effectively by or under the supervision of a qualified physical therapist.

Generally, range of motion exercises that are not related to the restoration of a specific loss of function but rather are related to the maintenance of function (see §271.1D2) do not require the skills of a qualified physical therapist.

The following conditions must be met: The services must be considered under accepted standards of practice to be a specific and effective treatment for the patient's condition.

Co-Treatment

503.3 Occupational Therapy Availability There may be instances where two or more disciplines are providing therapy services to the same patient. There may also be occasions where these services are duplicative. Your intermediary uses your documentation to determine if duplication exists. The following are some examples where there is not a duplication of services:

Transfers. Physical therapy instructs the patient in transfers to ascertain the level of safety with the techniques. Occupational therapy instructs and utilizes transfers as they relate to the performance of daily living skills, e.g., transfer from wheelchair to bathtub for bathing.

Pulmonary. Physical therapy teaches the patient an adapted breathing program. Occupational therapy carries the breathing retraining program into activities of daily living training.

Hip Fractures/Arthroplasties. Physical therapy instructs the patient in hip precautions and gait training. Occupational therapy carries out and reinforces the precautions when training the patient in activities of daily living, e.g., lower extremity dressing, toileting, and bathing.

CVA. Physical therapy utilizes upper extremity neurodevelopmental treatment (NDT) techniques to assist the patient in positioning the upper extremities on a walker and in gait training. Occupational therapy utilizes upper extremity (NDT) techniques to increase the functional use of upper extremities for dressing, bathing, grooming, and so on.

As with all rehabilitation services, your documentation must indicate a reasonable expectation that the patient will make material improvement within a reasonable period of time.

Professional Services. Services are sometimes performed by speech–language pathologists, occupational therapists, and physical therapists in concert with other health professionals. Services may be documented as performed by a team with each member performing unique roles. Do not document duplicate services. Clearly delineate roles. Services may include, but are not limited to the following example:

EXAMPLE

One professional assisting with positioning, adaptive self-help devices, inhibiting abnormal oromotor and/or postural reflexes while another professional is addressing specific exercises to improve oromotor control, determining appropriate food consistency form, assisting the patient in difficulty with muscular movements necessary to close the buccal cavity or shape food in the mouth in preparation for swallowing. Another professional might address a different role, such as increasing muscle strength, sitting balance, and head control.

Relate the documentation to either loss of function or potential for change. As with other conditions/disorders, the reasonableness and necessity of services must be evident in your documentation.

Include:

- Changes in condition or functional status;
- History and outcome of previous treatment for the same condition; or
- Any other information that would justify the start of care.

Even where a patient's full or partial recovery is not possible, a skilled service still could be needed to prevent deterioration or to maintain current capabilities.

When rehabilitation services are the primary services, the key issue is whether the skills of a therapist are needed. The deciding factor is not the patient's potential for recovery, but whether the services needed require the skills of a therapist or whether they can be carried out by non-skilled personnel (See §214.3.A.).

A service that is ordinarily considered non-skilled could be considered a skilled service in cases in which, because of special medical complications, skilled nursing or skilled rehabilitation personnel are required to perform or supervise it or to observe the patient. In these cases, the complications and special services involved must be documented by physicians' orders and nursing or therapy notes.

The existence of a plaster cast on an extremity generally does not indicate a need for skilled care. However, a patient with a preexisting acute skin problem, preexisting peripheral vascular disease, or a need for special traction of the injured extremity might need skilled nursing or skilled rehabilitation personnel to observe for complications or to adjust traction.

Whirlpool baths do not ordinarily require the skills of a qualified physical therapist. However, the skills, knowledge, and judgment of a qualified physical therapist might be required where the patient's condition is complicated by circulatory deficiency, areas of desensitization, or open wounds.

The importance of a particular service to an individual patient, or the frequency with which it must be performed, does not, by itself, make it a skilled service.

AUTHOR'S NOTE

However, if there are complicating comorbidities or the potential for decline, skilled services may be indicated on an inpatient, home health, or outpatient basis.

EXAMPLE

A primary need of a non-ambulatory patient may be frequent changes of position in order to avoid development of decubitus ulcers. However, since such changing of position does not ordinarily require skilled nursing or skilled rehabilitation personnel, it would not constitute a skilled service, even though such services are obviously necessary. However, if instruction to caretakers is needed for positioning and transfer training, the short-term skilled instruction, with appropriate documentation should be covered.

EXAMPLE

A patient has undergone peripheral vascular disease treatment including revascularization procedures (bypass) with open or necrotic areas of skin on the involved extremity. Skilled observation and monitoring of the vascular supply of the legs is required.

EXAMPLE

A patient has undergone hip surgery and has been transferred to an SNF. Skilled observation and monitoring of the patient for possible adverse reaction to the operative procedure, development of phlebitis, skin breakdown, or need for the administration of subcutaneous Heparin, is both reasonable and necessary, as well as rehabilitation services to regain function.

EXAMPLE

A patient has been hospitalized following a heart attack and, following treatment but before mobilization, is transferred to the SNF. Because it is unknown whether exertion will exacerbate the heart disease, skilled observation is reasonable and necessary as skilled mobilization and rehabilitation is initiated, until the patient's treatment regimen is essentially stabilized.

EXAMPLE

A frail 85-year-old man was hospitalized for pneumonia. The infection was resolved, but the patient, who had previously maintained adequate nutrition, will not eat or eats poorly. The patient is transferred to an SNF for monitoring of fluid and nutrient intake, assessment of the need for tube feeding and forced feeding if required. Observation and monitoring by skilled nursing personnel of the patient's oral intake is required to prevent dehydration. In order to remobilize the patient, skilled rehabilitation services to regain function are needed.

If a patient was admitted for skilled observation but did not develop a further acute episode or complication, the skilled observation services still are covered so long as there was a reasonable probability for such a complication or further acute episode. "Reasonable probability" means that a potential complication or further acute episode was a likely possibility.

Teaching and Training Activities

Teaching and training activities that require skilled nursing or skilled rehabilitation personnel to teach a patient how to manage his treatment regimen would constitute skilled services. Some examples are: gait training and teaching of prosthesis care for a patient who has had a recent leg amputation; teaching patients the use and care of braces, splints, and orthotics, and any associated skin care; and teaching patients the proper care of any specialized dressings or skin treatments.

According to the SNF Carriers Manual, available at www.cms.gov, the following are relevant to physical therapy. Please note that they are not distinctly different than in any other setting, and are therefore, included.

Direct Skilled Rehabilitation Services to Patients

Skilled Physical Therapy
General. Skilled physical therapy services must meet all of the following conditions:

- The services must be directly and specifically related to an active written treatment plan designed by the physician after any needed consultation with a qualified physical therapist.
- The services must be of a level of complexity and sophistication, or the condition of the patient must be of a nature that requires the judgment, knowledge, and skills of a qualified physical therapist;
- The services must be provided with the expectation, based on the assessment made by the physician of the patient's restoration potential, that the condition of the patient will improve materially in a reasonable and generally predictable period of time, or the services must be necessary for the establishment of a safe and effective maintenance program;
- The services must be considered under accepted standards of medical practice to be specific and effective treatment for the patient's condition; and
- The services must be reasonable and necessary for the treatment of the patient's condition; this includes the requirement that the amount, frequency, and duration of the services must be reasonable.

EXAMPLE 1

An 80-year-old, previously ambulatory, post-surgical patient has been bedbound for one week and, as a result, has developed muscle atrophy, orthostatic hypotension, joint stiffness, and lower extremity edema. To the extent that the patient requires a brief period of daily skilled physical therapy services to restore lost functions, those services are reasonable and necessary.

AUTHOR'S NOTE

Based on progress, this patient would probably qualify for continued services on a home health and possibly outpatient basis to return to independence.

EXAMPLE 2

A patient with congestive heart failure also has diabetes and previously had both legs amputated above the knees. Consequently, the patient does not have a reasonable potential to achieve ambulation, but still requires daily skilled physical therapy to learn bed mobility and transferring skills, as well as functional activities at the wheelchair level.

AUTHOR'S NOTE

If the patient has a reasonable potential for achieving those functions in a reasonable period of time in view of the patient's total condition, the physical therapy services are reasonable and necessary.

If the expected results are insignificant in relation to the extent and duration of physical therapy services required to achieve those results, the physical therapy would not be reasonable and necessary, and thus would not be covered skilled physical therapy services.

AUTHOR'S NOTE

The following are also excerpted from the Carrier Manual at www.cms.gov. They are found in the SNF guidelines, but are consistent for coverage for Medicare beneficiaries in other settings as well.

1. Application of Guidelines.
   Some of the more common physical therapy modalities and procedures are:
   a. Assessment.
      The skills of a physical therapist are required for the ongoing assessment of a patient's rehabilitation needs and potential. Skilled rehabilitation services concurrent with the management of a patient's care plan include tests and measurements of range of motion, strength, balance, coordination, endurance, and functional ability.
   b. Therapeutic Exercises.
      Therapeutic exercises that must be performed by or under the supervision of the qualified physical therapist, due either to the type of exercise employed or to the condition of the patient, constitute skilled physical therapy.
   c. Gait Training.
      Gait evaluation and training furnished a patient whose ability to walk has been impaired by neurological, muscular, or skeletal abnormality require

the skills of a qualified physical therapist and constitute skilled physical therapy if they reasonably can be expected to improve significantly the patient's ability to walk.

Repetitious exercises to improve gait, or to maintain strength, endurance, and assistive walking are appropriately provided by supportive personnel, i.e., aides or nursing personnel, and do not require the skills of a physical therapist. Thus, such services are not skilled physical therapy.

d. Range of Motion.

Only the qualified physical therapist may perform range of motion tests and, therefore, such tests are skilled physical therapy. Range of motion exercises constitute skilled physical therapy only if they are part of active treatment for a specific disease state which has resulted in a loss or restriction of mobility (as evidenced by physical therapy notes showing the degree of motion lost and the degree to be restored).

Range of motion exercises, which are not related to the restoration of a specific loss of function often may be provided safely by supportive personnel, such as aides or nursing personnel, and may not require the skills of a physical therapist. Passive exercises to maintain range of motion in paralyzed extremities that can be carried out by aides or nursing personnel would not be considered skilled care.

e. Maintenance Therapy.

The repetitive services required to maintain function sometimes involve the use of complex and sophisticated therapy procedures and, consequently, the judgment and skill of a physical therapist might be required for the safe and effective rendition of such services. (See §214.1.B.) The specialized knowledge and judgment of a qualified physical therapist may be required to establish a maintenance program intended to prevent or minimize deterioration caused by a medical condition, if the program is to be safely carried out and the treatment aims of the physician achieved. Establishing such a program is a skilled service.

EXAMPLE

A Parkinson's patient who has not been under a restorative physical therapy program may require the services of a physical therapist to determine what type of exercises are required for the maintenance of his present level of function. The initial evaluation of the patient's needs, the designing of a maintenance program which is appropriate to the capacity and tolerance of the patient and the treatment objectives of the physician, the instruction of the patient or supportive personnel (i.e., aides or nursing personnel) in the carrying out of the program, and such infrequent reevaluations as may be required, would constitute skilled physical therapy.

While a patient is under a restorative physical therapy program, the physical therapist should regularly reevaluate his condition and adjust any exercise program the patient is expected to carry out alone or with the aid of supportive personnel to maintain the function being restored. Consequently, by the time it is determined that no further restoration is possible (i.e., by the end of the last restorative session), the physical therapist will have already designed the maintenance program required and instructed the patient or supportive personnel in the carrying out of the program.

---

f. Ultrasound, Shortwave, and Microwave Diathermy Treatments.
These modalities must always be performed by or under the supervision of a qualified physical therapist and are skilled physical therapy.

g. Hot Packs, Infra-Red Treatments, Paraffin Baths, and Whirlpool Baths.
Heat treatments and baths of this type ordinarily do not require the skills of a qualified physical therapist. However, the skills, knowledge, and judgment of a qualified physical therapist might be required in the giving of

such treatments or baths in a particular case, e.g., where the patient's condition is complicated by circulatory deficiency, areas of desensitization, open wounds, fractures, or other complications.

Summary

All payers of physical therapy require that billing be completed on specific forms. However, most payers use a standard CMS 1500 form (some use UB forms) that includes only demographic information, with diagnosis codes, and CPT codes relating to the diagnosis, with the date(s) of service. If records are requested to support the claims, copies of all patient/client records for the dates of treatment are required in whatever format the provider PT uses at their facility. CMS, however, for Medicare beneficiaries, requires either the CMS 1500 form (see Appendix C) or the 700 series (see Appendix B) forms depending on the venue in which the services were rendered. For Medicare billing, there are specific documentation requirements that must be followed. Reimbursement can be denied for lack of compliance to the documentation regulations.

Regardless of the format for billing, attention must be paid to consistent terminology and the matching of all elements; billing dates, treatment dates and times, diagnostic codes (IDC-9), procedural codes (CPT), identified patient problems, established goals, interventions, initial examination results, all visit entries, and discharge information. All entries must indicate the necessity for skilled PT. If progress plateaus or stops at any point in the care, consideration must be made to discharge the patient. All care must be reasonable and necessary. The documentation content is the only supporting evidence of medical necessity and the justification of reasonable and necessary care.

Chapter 6 Review Questions

1. What are the advantages of using pre-made forms for documentation and billing purposes?

2. Provide four examples of terms that should be avoided in documentation.

3. Can Medicare be billed by the PT for restorative services? Defend your answer.

4. In order for PT services to be considered reasonable and necessary, what criteria have to be met?

5. What is co-treatment? Can more than one service bill for co-treatments? Explain your answer.

6. Compare and contrast certification and recertification in the Medicare context.

7. Under what circumstances is gait training skilled versus unskilled?

8. What constitutes an evaluation?

9. What is the difference between a CMS 1500 form and a CMS 700 form?

10. What are duplicate services? Provide examples of a procedure that might be considered duplicative unless the documentation indicates otherwise.

7

Legal Issues in the Medical Record

Introduction

"Effective patient care documentation is as important as the delivery of care itself."[19] The process of health information management by healthcare professionals presents challenges and legal responsibilities. In all documentation, physical therapy professionals must abide by professional standards, ethical codes, accreditation, and legal requirements in creating a permanent record of patient data.

Physical therapists are responsible for creating, maintaining, and disclosing patient care medical record information as dictated by law. Legally, the records created serve as the best evidence of the care rendered and whether the professional and legal standards of care was met or breached. For these reasons, physical therapists who document and collect patient-related health information need to understand medical record/health information law so that they can act responsibly in complying with applicable law and identify the need to obtain expert legal advice as applicable.

The significance of documenting patient care accurately, comprehensively, concisely, objectively, and in a reasonable time cannot be overemphasized. The consequences of altered, incomplete, or nonexistent records can be legally catastrophic. Practical application of risk management (prevention of any type of loss—financial or otherwise) and quality care must include proper documentation. The medical record frequently is the most important document available in defending against a claim of negligent or improper healthcare and is generally admissible at a trial.

Changing Environment

With respect to the constantly changing healthcare environment, the growth of managed care organizations, the use of technological advances, and the move toward primary care provision, therapists are assuming new duties in their roles as healthcare providers and in healthcare organization delivery systems.

With the dominance of managed care delivery, third-party payer reimbursement requires proper authorization from persons with little knowledge of the field of physical therapy. Therefore, therapists need to be effective advocates for their patients to ensure appropriate treatment. The need to document defensively is an important tool against allegations of substandard care and obtaining necessary authorization is vital to treat and receive payment. With the traditional fee-for-service process, practitioners enjoyed freedom in exercising autonomy in making decisions related to patient care. With the increased involvement of third-party payers, therapists disclose patient health information to the third-party payers who control the decisions regarding care issues, such as visit authorization. Working within the stringent allowances for treatment periods has been a challenge for clinicians.

Documentation cannot solve the dilemma of extending treatment for those whom have been terminated by third-party payers, but proper recording of patient care can still serve the patient in need of more treatment while protecting against risk of liability.

Medical Record as a Business and Legal Document

The medical record serves as a legal document with the purpose of providing substantive and objective evidence of care rendered when malpractice is alleged. The documentation forms a basis from which an expert witness can formulate an opinion as to whether acceptable standards of care were met. It also may provide substantive evidence of work or functional capacity in workers' compensation hearings and other administrative proceedings. Informed consents serve to protect healthcare providers and organizations by demonstrating evidence that a patient understood the risks and benefits of a procedure and made an informed decision to proceed with care. Inclusion in the documentation of patient's goals for therapy and their participation in the decision-making aspects of care, will verify patient autonomy. In cases where patients/clients have signed advanced directives, appropriate documentation protects providers who must carry out the directives.

Generally, laws, regulations, and standards contain requirements for medical recordation relevant to end-of-life decision making. The medical record should clearly detail pertinent information concerning the patient's decision and plan prior to the physician's order to withdraw or forego life-sustaining treatment.

Healthcare is a multi-trillion dollar industry. Routine documentation is mandatory and primary healthcare providers are required by legal, business, and ethical standards to record and safeguard clinically relevant patient history, examination and evaluative findings, and treatment-related information in patient health information records. The information may be entered electronically or manually, and the record maintained electronically or in hard copy for the time dictated by law.

State and federal laws, organizational policies and procedures, and customary practices in the setting, should be consulted to determine who can legally write patient health information in the medical record. The patient care record is a routinely generated business record that serves as the legal record of the nature, extent, and quality of care given the patient. As a result of this role, the medical record has both business and legal significance and as such serves to protect the patient and the professional.

The Medical Malpractice Crisis

Since the 1970s, there has been a "malpractice crisis" characterized by excessive numbers of lawsuits and verdicts in favor of patient/clients primarily against physicians and large organizations. Physical therapists are increasingly vulnerable with the expansion of professional practice into primary care, direct access, clinical specialization, and responsibilities delineated in *The Guide to Physical Therapist Practice* (APTA, 2001). Effective, systematic communication with patients/clients and other health professionals involved in care, with appropriate documentation, helps to reduce risk. Not only may accurate, complete, timely, and concise documentation save patient lives, writing incorporating these criteria may save a professional career. In an action for malpractice, the written treatment record may be the sole objective evidence of whether care to the patient was in compliance with acceptable standards or was substandard.

The Law

Statutes

Through law, relationships among private individuals, organizations, and government are defined and governed. The four primary sources of law are constitutions, statutes, administrative agencies, and court decisions. The U.S. Constitution is considered the supreme law of the land because it establishes and grants power to the three branches of federal government (legislative, executive, and judicial), and restricts actions of federal and state governments. The first ten amendments to the Constitution are called the Bill of Rights. The 14th Amendment places comparable due process requirements on state governments and assures equal protection under the law. With respect to hospitals and healthcare professionals, the constitutional right to privacy is often at issue.

Laws enacted by legislatures (U.S. Congress, state, and local legislatures) are called statutes. For situations in which federal and state law conflict, valid federal law supercedes. When state and local laws conflict, valid state law supercedes. Medical records laws are generally governed by state legislation and regulation. Applicable medical information provisions are found in laws for healthcare information confidentiality, healthcare provider licensure (practice), communicable diseases, child and elder abuse, peer review, and the dying process.

Administrative Rules and Regulations

The legislature (federal or state), commonly delegates authority to healthcare agencies to regulate and enforce laws because it lacks the time and expertise to address the complex issues involved. Courts interpret and determine whether statutes and regulations are constitutional and render decisions in matters not controlled by existing laws.

Professional Negligence

The legal bases for imposing liability on physical therapists are: professional negligence, breach of contract, strict product liability, strict liability, and intentional misconduct. Professional negligence or medical malpractice occurs when the delivery of patient care falls below the acceptable standard of care; minimal standards of ordinary, reasonable practitioners acting under similar circumstances. When a therapist performs or does not perform something during examination, evaluation, treatment, or follow-up, that other similarly situated therapists would not find acceptable, and harm comes to the patient, professional negligence exists. In pursuing a successful action for professional negligence, the injured party or plaintiff must prove by a preponderance of the evidence or that it is more likely than not that:

1. the therapist owed the patient a special duty of care;
2. the therapist failed to exercise that duty of care;
3. the violation of the standard of care caused physical and/or mental injury to the patient; and
4. the patient suffered legally recognizable money damages.

Patient Abandonment

When a healthcare provider unilaterally terminates a professional relationship with a patient inappropriately, legal abandonment occurs. Legal abandonment can be considered professional negligence or intentional misconduct. Legal abandonment occurs as a result of leaving a patient unattended temporarily, terminating service when a patient has not achieved rehabilitative goals, or terminating service if a patient's progress plateaued. Unilateral termination of the professional–patient relationship is legal when the patient voluntarily makes an informed election to end the relationship, or there is mutual agreement. The practitioner can only terminate the care unilaterally when the medical condition has resolved or therapy goals are met. If not, they can be at risk for inappropriate premature discharge. To avoid claims of unjustified, unilateral termination, physical therapists must carefully document all activities in the patient's care record.

When a third-party payer has pre-authorized a specific number of visits, the patient/client must be advised at the start of care. If the therapist decides to seek reconsideration for additional visits, care must be taken not to promise that it will be obtained. Additionally, if the therapist emphasizes the need for additional care and authorization is not granted for additional visits, the therapist may be held responsible for "abandoning" the patient/client if the patient believed additional care was needed. Alternatively, the therapist can offer the option of private pay. If the patient/client declines, this can be documented to avoid the appearance or accusation of abandonment.

If services are provided pro bono (free of charge) at the outset, physical therapists are held to the same standards of professional performance and abandonment regardless of the form of reimbursement.

Confidentiality, Privacy, and Access

Legislation in most states supports the patient–provider relationship and imposes a duty to guard against unauthorized disclosure on licensed health providers. The Health Insurance Portability and Accountability Act (HIPAA) of 1996, imposes a higher level of privacy and confidentiality on all providers of healthcare than ever before. The HIPAA privacy standards establish an individual's right to access their health information, provide limitations when access can be denied, and lists legal requirements for compilation and storage of patient medical information. (HIPAA restricts access to psychotherapy information compiled in anticipation of legal proceedings.) HIPAA also requires healthcare organizations to designate a privacy officer to oversee and implement all health information privacy policies and procedures because the standards in their entirety are complex.

Prior to the HIPAA privacy rule, there was no generally applicable federal legislation protecting confidentiality of medical or personal information. There was a lack of conformity of existing regulations governing access, use, and disclosure from state to state. Accrediting agencies, such as the Joint Commission on Accreditation of Healthcare Organizations, have also developed standards to assure security and confidentiality of the patient health data collected.

Computerization of patient information has enabled the immediate data exchange among authorized providers, payers, employers, and consumers both regionally and nationally. The use of electronic format in disclosing patient information is cost effective and promotes quality of patient care. However, computerized records create challenges in protecting patient privacy as a result of the continual lessening of release guidelines. It is also becoming increasingly difficult to determine who owns and is responsible for protecting against unauthorized access to the medical content.

In 2003, the healthcare provider owns the medical record, which may be released or accessed only in accordance with the law. The ownership of the medical record is less clearly that of only the individual provider in managed care settings where the individual providers are employees of larger healthcare organizations. Under Florida law, for example, the employer may be the record owner (Fla. Stat. Ch. 455.241).

Healthcare staff must access patient medical records for care reasons, administrative purposes, and defense against lawsuits. However, all staff are legally required to safeguard the confidentiality of the records and prevent unauthorized use of the information. Generally, facilities have established policies and procedures to ensure that confidentiality of health information is maintained.

Specific state laws allow reporting of patient health information without patient authorization when reporting vital statistics or matters affecting the public health, safety, or welfare. Some examples include reporting child abuse or neglect, presence of communicable diseases, and victims of violent crimes. Since these requirements vary among the states, knowledge and understanding of reporting requirements for the state in which the provider practices is a necessity.

To comply with HIPAA rules regarding disclosure, healthcare providers must obtain the patient's consent to access, use, or disclose personally identifiable health information for purposes of treatment, payment, and healthcare operations (TPO). Consent should be obtained when care is rendered and it ordinarily does not specify a date of termination or revocation of the consent. With patient consent, only that information minimally necessary to accomplish the intended purpose can be revealed.

Patient authorization is required for use or disclosure of information beyond the minimum necessary for treatment, payment, or support of healthcare operations.

The HIPAA privacy rule requires that healthcare providers and other covered entities must limit use, access, and disclosure to maintain patient privacy. Further, the same standard applies to use of information by individuals working for the facility. Any staff requiring access to the record should be identified in policies.

The HIPAA privacy rule, in general, requires that individuals have a right to a notice of privacy practice explaining how private health information will be used and disclosed. The notice should explain the individual's rights and covered entity's legal duties with respect to the private information. In most applications, patient consent must be obtained at the time the healthcare services are provided. According to HIPAA, the consent must be in plain language.

Protected health information under the privacy rule is expansive and includes information transmitted or maintained by electronic media or other form or medium. The privacy extends to any health information in any form or medium, including paper and oral forms. The privacy standard also refers to designated record sets: health records, billing records, and various claims records used to make decisions about individuals.

As with many rules, patients are free to waive their privilege to privacy and nondisclosure of health information. It is recommended that any such waiver be written. Healthcare providers and facilities may be subject to civil and criminal liability for disclosing patient health information that has not be authorized by the patient or required by law.

Because insurers and managed care organizations (MCOs) generally require patient information before making utilization review or reimbursement decisions, some states have laws or have adopted the National Association of Insurance Commissioners Insurance Information and Privacy Protection Model Act (NAIC Model Act), which requires that confidentiality of information be preserved and that disclosure is limited to particular circumstances.

Regardless of general laws, access to certain patient records, for example patients with alcohol and drug abuse problems, are expressly controlled by state and federal laws. Many states have special laws addressing staff access to records of mental health and AIDs patients. Only those staff with a need to know and directly involved in a patient's care are allowed access by law.

The Privacy Act of 1974 places restrictions on the type of information a federal agency may collect about citizens and legal aliens and limits how the information can be used (5 U.S.C. sect. 552a). The Act ensures that individuals can access and make copies of their records.

The constitutionally protected right to privacy is not absolute and is limited to violations by federal agencies and government contractors. Hospitals operated by the federal government and MCOs that provide health insurance to government employees are subject to the guidelines of the Act. Healthcare facilities that receive federal funding may be subject to the Act. Requested changes may be made to the information or explanation provided for denial of the request. Under certain circumstances, the Act permits the disclosure of information without consent.

The Freedom of Information Act (FOIA) of 1966 allows public access to information about the operations and decisions of federal administrative agencies. Specific categories of information are available to the public subject to nine specific exceptions. Of the noted exceptions, personnel and medical files are relevant to healthcare in that disclosure would violate rights to privacy. Requested records must be made available promptly and there are rules establishing when and where the records can be inspected and the fee for copying.

Laws permit the patient or patient representative to examine and copy the medical record. This requires a written request and payment of reasonable clerical costs for copying the record. State laws provide that records only need to be made available at reasonable times and places.

Responding to a Patient Request for Release of Health Information

There are many reasons a patient may request his or her records other than for a potential malpractice claim. It may be prudent and a good risk management procedure to meet with the patient and answer questions directly and in layperson's terms. This type of meeting may be the last effort to prevent a claim or litigation.

Copies of healthcare records and other patient health information should not be disclosed to third parties unless the patient authorizes the medical records release in a signed document. Therapists should request a copy of this release from a third-party payer prior to releasing a copy of the patient's record.

Generally, disclosure of the medical record of a minor requires authorization from one parent or legal guardian. Parents typically are permitted access to a child's medical information. Under certain circumstances, the minor may be able to authorize release of medical information.

The Internet is increasingly being used for transmission of clinical information. Every healthcare provider and organization should exercise care to maintain patient confidentiality. Policies and procedures should enforce confidentiality standards and ensure appropriate secure technology. The primary risks in using the Internet are related to unauthorized access and unauthorized disclosure of healthcare information. American Health Information Management Association (AHIMA) has developed guidelines for Internet use and security concerns. Healthcare providers using the Internet should comply with the AHIMA standards.

Legal Requirements for Medical Records

Record Security

It is important to safeguard medical records not only to protect patient confidentiality but also to prevent intentional alteration, removal, destruction, or falsification. It is HIPAA required to store records in a secure, restricted location; not to allow removal of the record from the premises unless court ordered; and to supervise patients and their representatives when examining the record.

Required Records

Healthcare providers must keep a medical record for each patient, according to proper record-keeping procedures. Failure to abide by this requirement may result in liability. Policies should designate the types of patient care information to be included in each patient record, the length of time for record retention, and the proper methods for destruction of the record.

Patient medical records consist of personal, financial, social, and medical data. Personal information contains identification information such as name, birth date, sex, marital status, next of kin, occupation, and physician name(s). Information about the patient's employer, health insurance carrier, types of insurance coverage and policy numbers, and Medicare and Medicaid numbers are considered financial and are used for billing purposes. The patient's race and ethnicity, family relationships, community activities, and information about lifestyle or court orders are considered social data. The continuous recordation of the history of treatment form the clinical record. This may consist of patient complaint(s), medical and family histories, results of physical or other medically related examinations, course of treatment, diagnosis and therapeutic orders, informed consent, clinical observations, progress notes, consultation reports, nursing notes, reports of diagnostic tests and procedures, and operative reports.

The medical record may be hand written, typed, or computer-generated, but should be consistent in format and content data for each discipline. The record should be a complete, accurate, and current account of the history, condition, and treatment of the patient, including outcomes and all other appropriate information in chronological order.

Content Requirements

The contents required to be included in patient healthcare records vary and generally depend on relevant state and federal laws and regulations, accreditation standards, organizational and system requirements, patient clinical settings and professional guidelines such as those contained in the *Guide to Physical Therapist Practice* (APTA, 2001).

Therapists should know the rules and regulations for record content as required by the state in which they work. With the advent of technology, access to state and federal regulations is available through the Internet.

Healthcare providers who participate in federal reimbursement programs must comply with the federal regulations for record maintenance, which may require a clinical record for each patient be maintained in accordance with professional standards, and to be promptly completed, filed, and retained [42 C.F.R. sect. 482.24 (hospitals); 42 C.F.R. sect. 418.74 (hospices); and 42 C.F.R. sect. 484.48 (home health agencies)]. In facilities participating with CMS compliance, specific criteria for record content must be met. Conditions for CMS records are similar for all settings in which Medicare beneficiaries receive physical therapy.

Accrediting organizations also impose maintenance standards for records. The Joint Commission requires the content of the health record in managed care facilities and hospitals to include: member identification, diagnoses, plan of care, medical history, appropriate physical examinations, immunization and screening status, results of treatments, procedures and tests, referrals or transfers to other practitioners, and evidence of advance directives. For home health accreditation, records must contain patient's height and weight, dietary restrictions, documentation as to suitability of home for services provided, documentation of patient and family education, and list of individuals and organizations involved in the patient's care, as well as the information required by federal regulation such as those for the Medicare program.

Most facilities have adopted formal written policies concerning the content of medical records. For PTs, it is good practice to adopt and follow the content criteria established in the APTA *Guide to Documentation* (See Appendix E) in conjunction with the most current applicable state, federal, and accreditation requirements associated with medical records. As laws change, it is important to monitor for new pertinent laws and regulations.

Formats

Practitioners should ensure that the content and format used for documentation of patient/client information is understood by others involved in the care of the patient. It is up to the facility, department, or therapists to determine which format is selected. Additionally, from an organizational perspective, there should be consistency in content and format within a department and between therapists. Quality Improvement (QI) or Quality Assurance (QA) initiatives should ensure that content is complete and appropriate to ensure the record will serve all identified purposes (See Chapter 12). Regardless of the format selected, the content should be objective in nature with all information matching and relevant. The necessity of the need for skilled intervention should be clear based on identified problems, planned interventions, and relevance of functional goals or outcomes.

Interestingly, written goals represent professional judgment and not necessarily a guarantee or warranty of a specific therapeutic result. Legally, patient intervention goals are generally not actionable. However, actual communication of therapeutic promises may create contractual obligations to patients and create legal liability if not achieved.

Problems, Errors, and Practice

Problems with documentation can have serious legal ramifications. Therefore, it is important that therapists familiarize themselves with common errors and the recommendations for averting adverse consequences. Please also refer to Chapter 6 for more information.

Illegibility

Illegibility is a common documentation problem and may result in inability to translate patient care information. The solution is for therapists to write legibly, print, type, or utilize alternative documentation systems not based on handwritten notation. Additionally, the record must be complete. This is reinforced in the Medicare guidelines, which require that all entries be legible and complete [42 C.F.R. sect. 482.24(c)].

Patient's Full Name

The patient's full name and identifying information should be on every page. Failure to correctly identify a patient receiving care is negligence and can lead to liability. When the record is copied, the lack of patient identification on any page can result in inappropriate filing or loss of information.

Date and Time of Patient Care

The date and usually the time of patient care should be included in all records. This will support time billed for that patient and can be used as evidence in any patient dispute regarding date and time of visit.

Standard Forms and Formats

Standard forms and formats that are universally understood by other providers in the same facility or network should be used. Standardization helps to ensure appropriate content and consistency.

Indelible Black or Blue Ink

Indelible black or blue ink should be used for documenting patient care to prevent tampering with entries, especially in the advent of legal action. However, the facility must determine which color will be used by policy and to ensure uniformity.

In the event the pen runs out of ink while documenting, a therapist must complete the note. If another ink color is used, an explanation in parentheses should precede the second part of the patient note stating that the original pen ran out of ink. This parenthetical explanation should be initialed. This procedure is necessary to avoid implications of spoilage of records in a potential lawsuit.

Computerized entries should be saved automatically to prevent subsequent loss or alteration of patient content.

Blank Spaces

Blank spaces or lines are unacceptable in the record, as blanks may infer lack of completeness or create the potential to add information. Therapists should use each line to document care, leaving no spaces between lines or by putting diagonal lines through large empty spaces.

Signatures

Signatures (or initialing patient care corrections or flowsheets) on entries are required for authentication purposes and to acknowledge legal and ethical responsibility for the information contained in the entry. Entries should bear legible legal signatures followed by professional title to demonstrate a skilled professional rendered care. In most states, computer signatures constitute legal signatures, but the therapist should seek legal counsel for verification. Licensure number is recommended.

Error Correction

Error correction, commonly consists of a single line drawn through the erroneous content, initialed, and dated, preferably with the time. The most important rule is not to hide the mistake by whiting it out, scratching it out, blacking it out, or writing over it. The addition of the words "error" or "mistake" are controversial and create an image of sloppy patient care in a malpractice setting.

Addendum

Addendums can be made or added to the patient record and should always contain the date of the addendum. Amendments made at the patient's request should be included as an addendum with a notation explaining that the change was made at the patient's request. Patient amendments that are deemed inappropriate should be discussed with the patient. Generally, if the requested change is not made by the facility, it may be a good idea to permit the individual to insert a statement of disagreement in the record. Some states allow this procedure provided notice of change or statement is given to designated persons within certain time periods.

Intentional alteration of a medical record or writing an incorrect record may subject a provider to statutory sanctions, including license revocation. Altering or falsifying a chart to obtain Medicare or state health reimbursement is a crime under federal law punishable with substantial fine or imprisonment [42 U.S.C. sect. 1320a-7b(a)].

**Acceptable
Abbreviations**

Acceptable abbreviations save time and facilitate accurate communication. However, problems arise when abbreviations have more than one meaning or are not widely known. Physical therapists should only use abbreviations that have been approved or are universally disseminated. If providers relying on unintelligible abbreviations cause injury to patient, then both the author and reader of the erroneous information may be liable for malpractice (See Appendix A).

**Improper Spelling
and Grammar and
Wordiness**

Improper spelling and grammar and wordiness create a negative impression of practitioner carelessness that contributes to findings of liability. All entries should be as accurate and concise as possible to avoid confusion or discrepancy.

Orders

Illegible PT orders must be clarified before seeing the patient or carrying out the orders. Therapists should document any inquiries and physician responses regarding ambiguities in diagnostic and treatment orders. State laws, policies of the facility, accreditation standards, and customary practices govern whether care is elicited under verbal orders. For most therapists, laws require written referrals. Physical therapists who evaluate patients under verbal referral orders should require the referring physician or other provider to promptly authenticate the orders in writing, preferably within 24 hours. This practice will enhance communication and protect both the referring physician and the therapist. Policies related to verbal orders should require that only personnel qualified to understand physician orders be authorized to receive and transcribe them. In direct access states, therapists should know the laws regarding the need, if any, to refer to a physician. Written orders are preferable because they create fewer chances for error.

**Documentation
Timeliness**

Documentation should occur as closely as possible to when the care is rendered. The longer the time between the care and the note is written, the less accurate it will be. Untimely documentation that results in prolonged care or patient discomfort is professional negligence and gives opposing attorneys opportunity to challenge the accuracy of the content. It is also unethical to document care before it is given. In the event a late entry into the medical records must be made, for example when the chart is unavailable, it should be designated as an "addendum" or "follow-up entry." From the legal perspective, timeliness of medical record entries is important. Late entries mean that the records are incomplete for a period of time. Transcribed or dictated entries should be received within 24 hours.

**Identification of
Information Sources**

Identification of information sources must be provided. Failing to denote another practitioner's responsibility for clinical information provided may result in legal liability solely to the writer of the note and leads to misinterpretations as to who is responsible for patient care. If a primary care provider receives and documents clinical information regarding an adverse change in patient status, the provider is obligated to re-examine the patient expeditiously and should document accordingly to reduce legal liability for inappropriate monitoring of the patient.

**Blame or
Disparaging
Comments**

Blame or disparaging comments should not appear in the record, unless the writer is willing to risk potential actions for defamation. However, statements made by patients must be entered into medical records in quotations. Before documenting a patient statement that appears contradictory to the patient's self-interest, the therapist should have the patient confirm the statement. In such a situation, it is advisable to have a witness and ethically, the statement must be documented in the patient record when is contains clinically pertinent information.

**Objective and
Specific Findings**

Objective and specific findings should be documented, whereas subjective findings or opinions should not. It is recommended that therapists avoid writing ambiguous statements such as "appears" or is "apparently" should be avoided. For example, ROM WNL (range of motion with normal limits) does not tell the reader what joints were examined and is, therefore, not sufficient.

Informed Consent

Informed consent for examination and treatment must be included, preferably as a separate form. However, it can be included by the therapist as a statement. Generally, the law requires that the patient be given sufficient information concerning the nature and risks of the recommended and alternative treatments to make an educated decision. In this way, the consent given is informed consent. The general rule is that if consent is not given, the patient is not serviced. However, the patient must be competent to make an appropriate decision based on the information received. In some circumstances, such as under emergencies and compulsory treatments, the law supercedes a patient's decision and care is given.

The Patient Self-Determination Act, effective December 1, 1991, codifies a patient's common law right to control their healthcare decisions and binds all facilities and providers participating in Medicare and Medicaid programs. The Act ensures that patients are educated to make "informed decisions" and have rights to make "advanced directives." The Act respects ethical rights of persons to make autonomous decisions about their bodies. In accordance with this law, facilities and organizations should require written informed consent from patients, including written policies and procedures protecting patient rights and documentation of whether a patient executed advanced directives.

A well-written, properly executed consent form is strong evidence that informed consent was given, although it is not legally conclusive. To be a legally effective consent form, the document should be signed voluntarily, indicate that the procedure performed is the same consented to, and demonstrate that the consenting person understood the nature of the procedure, the risks, and probable consequences. This can be done with a short or long form. The short form is generalized and does not contain specific risks and benefits. It is advisable to supplement the short form by writing detailed notes regarding risks and benefits discussed in the patient medical record. The long form includes a detailed description of the medical condition, proposed procedure, consequences, risks, and alternatives. The danger in using this form is that providers rely and may substitute the form rather than explain the information to the patient to assure understanding.

Generally, a person's consent constitutes authorization for a particular practitioner to perform a procedure so deviation from that authorization may invalidate the consent. Further, refusal of consent to treatment by a certain practitioner removes that practitioner from engaging in the treatment.

For situations in which adequacy of information given is disputed, courts will apply standards of the reasonable physician and the reasonable patient. The more modern approach is to apply the reasonable patient standard, wherein the physician's duty to provide information is determined by the information needs of the patient, not the professional practice.

Persons with difficulties understanding English must have the form translated. Healthcare providers servicing multiple cultural and ethnic populations should have consent forms in primary languages. It is usually sufficient to have a form translated orally. It is important to have the translator certify that the form and discussion of the procedure have been translated for the patient.

For minors, parent or guardian consent must be obtained before treatment is given. If the minor needs emergency treatment, a statute gives the minor the right to consent, or it is court or otherwise legally ordered. Legally, either parent can give effective consent for treatment except when parents are legally separated or divorced, at which time the consent of the custodial parent is typically required unless there is an agreement requiring both to consent. A provider can rely on the parent(s) to tell them who has authority to consent to the minor's care.

Special consent requirements beyond informing as to risks and benefits are needed when patients undergo experimental treatments or participate in clinical studies. Federal, state, and local laws impose strict requirements for obtaining patient consent and should be consulted.

When a patient's condition changes significantly, the original consent may no longer be valid and a new consent should be obtained. Patient refusal of consent and withdrawal of consent for treatment should be documented and the physician notified.

Theories of Consent There are two theories of consent violations. One theory is based on the common law development of battery or violation of an individual's right to be free from harmful or offensive touching. Another theory is based on negligence whereby patients consent to procedures without having sufficient information to make an informed decision.

Refusal of Consent Refusal of Consent is the legal right of competent adults to refuse medical treatment. Legally, courts have upheld these decisions despite the basis of the refusal. It is advisable to seek the advice of legal counsel for situations in which the refusal is a serious threat to health and endangers the patient's life.

When a patient refuses to sign the consent form but is willing to give consent orally, the fact of oral consent and the reason for refusal to sign the form should be documented on the consent form, along with the witnessed signature, and placed in the medical record.

Home Instructions/Independent Exercise Instructions/Instructions

Home instructions, home exercise programs, independent exercise programs and the like must be documented, copies maintained, and preferably contain the patient/client or responsible party's signature, indicating that they have received and understand them.

Standardized programs should be kept as part of clinical procedures manuals. As part of the documentation, the therapist should include that the patient, family, or other understands, safely carries out, and is responsibly complying with home programs of care. All precautions or limitations to activities and follow-up instructions must be documented. Lack of follow-up could be construed as actionable abandonment.

Noncompliance

Noncompliance, missed appointments, and refusal of care or to comply with given recommendations must be documented. The documentation should be objective, including specific times and dates of violations and circumstances/descriptions of noncompliance. If a patient fails to comply and goals are not met or they suffer harm, contributory negligence may be applicable.

Incidence or Occurrence Reports

Incidence or occurrence reports should not be included in the record or identified. It is important to objectively document the incident in the record and obtain quality care for any injuries. Risk management must be notified in order to protect the facility against unwarranted liability and educate to prevent similar future incidents. Incident reports preserve memories of incidents. Since the reports are considered more administrative in nature and purpose, they are maintained separately from the record.

Countersignature

Countersignature is expected for student documentation and recommended in the *APTA Guide to Physical Therapist Practice*. The reason the note must be cosigned is to authenticate the note and make it legally acceptable. The need for a countersignature legally is to assure that a professional has reviewed the note, and if appropriate, to indicate approval of action taken by another practitioner. The person who countersigns has the authority to evaluate the entry and typically has more experience or has higher training than the person making the entry. Countersignatures permit delegation of responsibility. Providers who countersign another's notes should carefully proofread the note before cosigning. The countersignature imposes legal responsibility for the information contained in the note. Incomplete or inaccurate notes should not be countersigned until corrected appropriately. Once countersigned by a physical therapist, the physical therapy student's note is legally adopted by the supervising therapist as his or her own note causing him or her to share the legal responsibility with the student for what is written in the note. Without evidence of that supervision inferred by countersignature, a student might be held as violating and engaging in the unlicensed practice of physical therapy.

Authentication

Authentication and signature is made by the provider who delivers the care. Handwritten signatures were traditionally required. More recently, rubber stamps and computer key signatures are accepted and permitted by some states, and computer or electronic signatures are allowed by state and federal authorities.

The Center for Medicare and Medicaid (CMS) requires authentication of each entry for Medicare participation. CMS does allow authentication by computer, but not all entities allow this type of "auto-authentication." Failure to obtain a physician's signature to the record in its final form constitutes deficiency (BNA Health Law Reporter, October 21, 1993).

AUTHOR'S NOTE

Rubber stamp signatures are not allowed on Medicare documentation.

Record Retention and Destruction

Therapists should check for applicable statutory and regulatory requirements dictating retention in their state. The general period for retention of medical records varies and should minimally cover the statute of limitations or period within which a party may bring a lawsuit. If participating under Medicare, retention of the original record or legally reproduced form must be for a period of at least five years. About half of the states require that original medical records be preserved for ten years. Some facilities require record retention beyond the statute of limitations, including rules for deceased patients.

The statute of limitations on contract and tort actions should also determine how long to keep records. Although most lawsuits brought by minors are done soon after the incident causing the injury, therapists should retain the records until a minor reaches majority and for an additional time equal to the state statute of limitations for tort actions. Generally, the medical record of a minor should be kept until the patient reaches the age of majority (18 or 21 depending on the state) plus the statute of limitations. For example for a state in which majority is 21 years and the statute of limitations for torts is two years, records should be preserved for 23 years.

For medical research purposes, it is advisable to establish a long retention period for records. When research involves experimental or innovative patient care procedures, records should be preserved for extended periods of time, typically 75 years.[20] This means that space for storage must be designated and recordation be in a format that will withstand this time. Storage of medical records on computers may be governed by licensure or accreditation laws, federal programs, or rules of evidence associated with admissibility of copies of patient records at trial.

The American Health Information Management Association (AHIMA) has established record retention guidelines to aid organizations in determining how well they measure up to industry standards. These guidelines include: ensuring availability of patient information for continued care; legal requirements; research, education, and other legitimate uses; developing a retention schedule for patients, physicians, researchers, and other user needs; legal, regulatory, and accreditation requirements; specifying what information is saved, for what time period, and how to store the information; establishing compliance programs addressing all types of documentation gen erated from employee training, hot lines, internal investigations, audits, modifications to compliance programs, and self-disclosures; retaining documentation for sufficient time to prove compliance with applicable federal and state laws and regulations; and developing policies with legal advice.

AHIMA's recommended minimum time periods for which patient health records be kept are:

- Patient health records (adults): 10 years after most recent encounter
- Patient health records (minors): Age of majority plus statute of limitations
- Diagnostic images: 5 years
- Disease index: 10 years
- Fetal heart monitor records: 10 years after infant reaches majority
- Master patient index: Permanently
- Operative index: 10 years
- Register of births: Permanently
- Register of deaths: Permanently
- Register of surgical procedures: Permanently

Courts have held facilities liable for an independent act of breaching their duty to make and maintain medical records and allowed an action to continue when a plaintiff had insufficient evidence to sustain a medical malpractice action because the patient health record could not be produced.[22]

The patient-health information records may be destroyed in accordance with state statute when the retention period expires or the record has been copied onto microfilm or computer, or otherwise converted into readable form. Some states require that an abstract of pertinent information in the medical record be created before destruction. Large facilities generally contract with a commercial enterprise for destruction of records. It is important that such an agreement contain terms dealing with the method of destruction, safeguards protecting confidentiality of information, indemnification, and certification that the records have been properly destroyed. Failure to apply a uniform policy to all records may result in a jury's interpretation that if the records were available, they would reveal that a patient received substandard care.

Medicare

The conditions relevant to participation in the Medicare program require medical records remain confidential. These conditions apply to various types of facilities including hospitals, long-term care facilities, home health agencies, substance abuse agencies, and hospices.

Disclosure of Medical Information for Research Purposes

Many states as well as the federal government have laws providing for disclosure of patient information for research projects, especially regarding research using human subjects. Most facilities have established Institutional Review Boards (IRB) that evaluate research protocol, protect the confidentiality of the information obtained, decide whether the research will benefit society, and determine whether adequate safeguards exist to protect the human study subjects placed at risk. With new HIPAA laws, it is required to obtain written patient authorization for any release of the medical record.

Special Documentation Concerns

Celebrity Patients

Special care to protect the patient health information records of celebrity patients may be challenging since the personalities are often subject to the close scrutiny of the news media. Some facilities have established policies and procedures to assess the need for anonymity, omit the patient name from the record or replace it with an alias or code name and maintain the record in a special secure file.

Hostile Patients

Hostile patients are more likely to take legal action in the event of rendered problematic or perceived problematic healthcare. It is recommended to create a detailed medical record that leaves little ambiguity regarding the medical care given the patient. Avoid inserting derogatory comments about the patient's behavior in the record, including only objective descriptions and quotes from the patient. Negative remarks may be used in litigation to prove bad faith on behalf of the practitioner.

Recording Indicators of Child or Elder Abuse

Documentation in suspected situations of abuse should be detailed and objective containing a description of all relevant findings. This is important as the documentation may be used for determination of abuse. The results of any assessments and testing should be included as well as a detailed history and identities of interviewers or other caregivers or family of the patient.

Durable Power of Attorney for Healthcare

Most states have adopted the Uniform Durable Power of Attorney that permits an agent of a disabled or incompetent person to make healthcare decisions on behalf of the patient. This document is more flexible than a living will, which is limited to when the patient is terminally ill or permanently unconscious. The durable power of attorney can be used whenever a patient is unable to communicate a choice regarding a health decision and is not limited to specific life-sustaining measures.

Do-Not-Resuscitate Orders

It is common practice to document in writing "Do not resuscitate" (DNR) or "No CPR" in the orders for patient treatment. Additionally, an appropriate consent form or refusal of treatment form should be signed by the patient, patient representative, or family member. It should be prominently displayed in the record so it is common knowledge.

Disagreeing Opinions Among Staff

All healthcare providers have the duty to take reasonable actions to safeguard the lives of their patients. Using professional judgment, a PT may encounter a situation in which it is necessary to clarify or object to physician orders or inform the physician of contraindications to treatment. Documentation of professional disagreements should be done in a manner that is objective, factual, nonjudgmental, and could not be used as evidence against the physician or institution in a negligence lawsuit. For example, is it not appropriate to write, "Dr. Joe is negligent again or the order is incorrect . . ." Most facilities will have policies and procedures for documenting professional differences of opinion.

Special Disclosures

Records Sought by Managed Care Organizations (MCO)

MCOs often need access to patient health information to monitor discharge planning, case management, utilization review, and credentialing of physicians. Requests for access are often established by way of policies and procedures to reduce liability for negligent access. These policies typically adopt applicable laws relating to keeping confidentiality of patient information.

Records Sought by Law Enforcement

The general rule is that healthcare providers and organizations should not release medical records or other patient health information to requesting law enforcement agencies without written authorization of the patient. Unless there is statutory authority, court order, or subpoena, the police have no authority to examine medical records.

Legal Issues Related to Improper Disclosure

Healthcare providers and facilities may be subject to civil and criminal liability for disclosing patient health information that has not been authorized by the patient or required by law. State statutes and regulations provide for criminal and professional disciplinary sanctions. State laws and common law usually allow wronged individuals to file civil suits and seek recovery of damages.

Causes of Action for Releasing Information Without Authorization

In order to sue successfully, a patient must be able to prove the elements of the legal cause of action. The legal theories pertinent to medical information liability are: defamation, invasion of privacy, and breach of confidentiality. A suit for defamation is typically based on common law and must prove: (1) a false and defamatory statement was made about the patient; (2) the statement was published to a third party; (3) the publishing party knew the statement was false or acted with reckless disregard of its truth or falsity; and (4) injury was caused by the statement or the statement by nature was harmful. If accusing invasion of privacy, the patient must show evidence of the improper disclosure of patient information. Another legal theory often governed by state statute and used by patients to sue healthcare providers who disclose medical record information is breach of confidentiality, or breach of physician–patient privilege. Generally, a violation of this confidentiality results in liability to the patient for damages caused by the disclosure that may have resulted in the deterioration of a marriage, loss of a job, and suffering of emotional distress.

Medicare Disclosure

Section 4311 of the Balanced Budget Act of 1997 requires that if a Medicare beneficiary submits a written request to a health services provider for an itemized statement for any Medicare item or service provided to that beneficiary, the provider must furnish this statement within 30 days of the request. The law also states that a health services provider not furnishing this itemized statement may be subject to a civil monetary penalty of up to $100 for each unfulfilled request. Since most institutional health practices have established an itemized billing system for internal accounting procedures as well as for billing other payers, the furnishing of an itemized statement should not pose any significant additional burden.

30-Day Period to Furnish Statement You will furnish to the individual described above, or duly authorized representative, no later than 30 days after receipt of the request, an itemized statement describing each item or service provided to the individual requesting the itemized statement.

Risk Management

Computerized or Electronic Medical Records

The trend in medicine is to grow with increasing use and reliance on technology. The methods of maintaining patient medical records in paper files with eventual transfer to microfilm for safekeeping is changing. Most providers use computers, computer networks, facsimile machines, and optical scanning and storage equipment to create, transmit, store, and retrieve patient healthcare information. Although computerization enhances the quality of patient care, there are risks related to maintaining confidentiality of the information and complex legal issues regarding the duties and rights of providers. Electronic data exchange from the numbers of computer links and electronic fund transfers has opened up the doors to potential healthcare fraud. The laws are not keeping pace with the advances in technology and there is very little legal precedent in the area. Licensure laws and regulations and Medicare and accreditation standards require providers and facilities to safeguard records and protect against unauthorized access. The legal confidentiality obligations are the same for electronic and paper-based systems. Most legislative protections governing confidentiality of patient health information only apply when the medical record data identifies the patient. Therefore, cleansed data may be used with very few restrictions.

There are legal questions regarding which state's law would apply to medical record information transmitted across state lines. Similarly, computerization of patient data increases risk of unauthorized disclosure. One violation of a computer system's security could result in numerous disclosures and potentially catastrophic liability since a system can access, copy, and transmit substantial numbers of records in short times. Therefore, safeguards must be built into the systems.

Electronic Claims

Standards for processing of health claims electronically have been established under the Health Insurance Portability and Accountability Act of 1966 (HIPAA) and mandate compliance.

Telemedical Records

The delivery of healthcare services from a distance using interactive telecommunications and computer technology is called telemedicine. The practice of using electronic signals to communicate medical information generates legal issues regarding accuracy from distortion of data, confidentiality, and security of health information. Airwaves are not secure and the confidentiality of patient health information cannot be guaranteed. Presently, there are very few legislative or accreditation requirements pertaining to the creation or maintenance of telemedical records. Because there are so few statutory or regulatory guidelines, all relevant standards should be followed.

Electronic Mail

Electronic mail (e-mail) is increasingly used to transmit sensitive patient health information. Although the modes of e-mail transmission have occurred at a rapid pace, the implementation of related technological safeguards have not developed at a similar pace and are less than adequate, creating more challenges for keeping confidentiality and security of medical records. Providers who send electronic messages must be aware to exercise caution when transmitting patient information to avoid compromising the integrity of the data and to prevent a breach of patient confidentiality. Title III of the Omnibus Crime Control and Safe Streets Act of 1968, commonly known as the federal wiretapping law, provides protection against improper interception of electronic communications, such as e-mail, and imposes civil and criminal liabilities on violators.

If a healthcare provider uses e-mail, it is important to develop policies and procedures addressing recording, retention, and destruction of the communications. E-mail communications should be included in patient medical records and follow the guidelines of documentation.

Medical Records in Legal Proceedings

As stated previously, patient treatment records provide clinical information about the patient to the various healthcare providers involved in that patient's care. As a business record, it justifies to third-party payers reimbursement for services provided, allows for monitoring of quality patient care, sets forth needs for risk management, and provides a basis for clinical research and educational training. Legally, the records protect the patients, healthcare providers and support staff. In litigation proceedings, the records may be the only written record of what transpired. As such, it could be effective in a positive defense against a claim of professional negligence or be the reason for an unfavorable decision against a provider. Failure to create or maintain the records is a breach of the duty owed the patient. If a breached duty results in a patient injury, then actionable malpractice may ensue.

Intentional failure to maintain records, or spoliation, is typically a criminal matter of fraud and obstruction of justice. A charge of spoliation can result in suspension or revocation of licensure and imposition of a fine. Healthcare providers must resist the urge to correct records that appear obviously erroneous. Changes to a record should be implemented in a manner as previously described. It is not difficult to spot an altered patient care entry. Common signs indicating alteration include: differences in handwriting, use of different writing instruments, erasures and/or obliteration or correction liquid, and non-uniform crowding of words particularly between lines or in margins. Similarly, signs of rewritten patient care entries may include: differences in paper type, binder holes or other markings that do not match the rest of the record, date and/or time discrepancies, subsequent entries that seem out of context or confusing, findings not known at the time, and handwriting style or quality inconsistent with the writer. To avert dangers of spoliation, facility risk managers routinely segregate original patient records involving patients in litigated claims.

Defense: Use of Health Records in Judicial Proceedings

Patient health records containing relevant information are usually admissible into evidence in judicial proceedings when someone is involved in the legal action. Under these circumstances, a court order by way of a subpoena duces tecum, is issued to require production of the medical information. State regulations governing court procedure indicate whether original or copies of the health records will suffice. A records custodian will need to testify as to the authenticity of any records produced.

The U.S. Legal System

Laws define specific relationships and are classified as public or private. Public laws involve relationships between individuals or businesses and the government and define, regulate, and enforce respective rights of the parties. For example, Medicare is public law and involves the government in its relationship providing health insurance for individuals. In comparison, private law involves rules and legal principles defining rights and duties between individuals and/or private businesses. Private laws apply in matters involving contracts or torts such as malpractice. There are four sources of public and private laws: constitutions, statutes, administrative law, and judicial decisions.

The U.S. Constitution defines and establishes the powers of the legislative, executive, and judicial branches of government. It also includes 26 amendments, the first ten comprising the Bill of Rights. Additionally, every state has a constitution, which is regarded as the highest law of the state but subordinate to the U.S. Constitution. Statutes are laws enacted by state legislatures and U.S. Congress. Accordingly, Medicare and HIPAA are statutes since they were enacted by the U.S. Congress.

Administrative rules and regulations are developed by administrative agencies to which Congress has given powers. For example, Congress has directed the Secretary of Health and Human Services to promulgate rules to carry out the intent of HIPAA. Judicial decisions interpreting the Constitution and statutes form a major source of law and serve as a primary source for private law.

Legal Proceedings   Lawsuits against healthcare providers are brought by plaintiffs who file complaints against an individual or company called the defendant. The next phase of the litigation is discovery, at which time medical records are often utilized to determine the strength of the opposing party's case. In depositions, a subpoenaed individual may be required to testify that health records were compiled in the normal course of business and have not been altered in any manner. Alternatively, individuals in positions as custodian of records will be subpoenaed to produce health records and other patient information. At trial, the medical records often are entered into evidence. Should a verdict or court decision be appealed, medical records that were admitted into evidence at trial may be reviewed by an appellate court. If a PT is deposed as part of a legal action, they will be asked a series of questions. It is always best to answer with only the content read from the record. The PT should not "try to remember."

Professional Liability

Medical malpractice refers to the professional liability of healthcare providers involved in the delivery of patient care. Professional liability may arise from breach of contract, intentional tort, and negligence theories.

The provider–patient relationship is established by either an express or an implied contract. Under either contract, an expectation of the scope of duty arises from the relationship, whereby the healthcare provider agrees to diagnose and/or treat the patient in accordance with standards of acceptable practice and to continue treating until the natural termination of the relationship, such as patient gets well or dies, mutual agreement to terminate, patient terminates, or healthcare provider withdraws from providing care. When the provider–patient relationship exists, failure to diagnose or treat using reasonable care and skill may give the patient cause to sue for breach of contract.

Healthcare providers are often held liable when they intentionally harm a person under the legal theory of tort. Intentional torts are wrongful acts that result in injury to another.

Negligence occurs when a healthcare provider commits a wrongful act by failing to do what another prudent reasonable healthcare provider would do under similar circumstances. Other causes of action against healthcare providers may include assault and battery, defamation, invasion of privacy, wrongful disclosure of confidential information, and abandonment.

Risk Management

AHIMA has published guidelines on health information management, health record documentation, and content based on the practice setting. To reduce risk, all facilities providing patient care should have policies ensuring uniformity of content and format of healthcare records based on applicable accreditation standards, federal and state regulations, payer requirements, and professional practice standards. In order to meet legal requirements, many guidelines should be followed, including systematic organization of health records to facilitate retrieval and compilation of information and quantitative and qualitative analysis of health records to confirm that state law, regulation, or healthcare facility licensure standards are upheld as related to documentation.

Computerized, Photographic, and Videotaped Patient Care Records

Increasingly more facilities are using computers to record patient data. The electronic records, however, pose a challenge to preserving patient confidentiality and temptations to alter or erase prior patient entries. Therefore, facilities must develop safeguards to protect access and unauthorized alteration.

Photographic documentation is also used by PTs to memorialize before and after treatments. The photographic evidence must be preserved in accordance with statutory retention requirements. Copying of photographs is more expensive and more time-consuming than paper, although computer scanning may reduce the cost.

Video documentation memorializing patient status and treatment is also used by physical therapists. Provided the videotape meets certain legal standards, it may be admitted into evidence if needed. Videotapes must be retained in accordance with statutory requirements. Photography or videotaping typically requires explicit written informed consent.

Special Circumstances Requiring Documentation/ Sexual Assault and Battery

It is important to obtain and safeguard results of examinations and care given victims of sexual assault or battery. Most facilities have written policies addressing recordation, storage, and transfer of patient health information to law enforcement authorities. Any statements made by a victim should be included in "quotes" in the documentation and may be admissible in a future court proceeding. Records of sexual assault patients should be maintained separate from the general patient care records. Facility policies and appropriate laws should be followed regarding reporting.

Documentation of Patient Restraint Use

Providers must document certain things before using physical restraints (or pharmacology) on patients. This requirement resulted from the danger of misuse and neglect related to the use of such restraints, especially in skilled nursing facilities. Practitioners must document clinical justification (patient behaviors) for using restraints by including documentation demonstrating that less restrictive alternatives were inadequate, other health providers have been consulted and that the patient's physical and mental conditions have been considered. The potential for harm must be included if the patient/client goes without restraints. Documentation and policy for the use of physical restraints must be consistent with federal and applicable state laws.

Reimbursement and Documentation

Documentation requirements for reimbursement are generally administratively controlled and constantly change. It is important for therapists to familiarize themselves on an ongoing basis with applicable requirements. Legal issues involve whether the documentation constitutes larceny (theft) by fraudulent or deceptive practices. Healthcare fraud occurs when there is an untruthful representation of a material fact. Billing for services not rendered, waivers of patient copayments and deductibles under Medicare Part B, violations of anti-kickback and self-referral laws, over utilization or unbundling of services, upcoding, or miscategorizing coding to enhance payments by third-party payers, if done knowingly, can result in an allegation of fraud. Inadequate patient care documentation may support or create a claim for fraud leading to liability with the Department of Health and Human Services (HHS). The penalties for reimbursement fraud range from civil fines to criminal convictions, administrative penalties, exclusion as Medicare and Medicaid providers or other third-party payer systems, suspension or revocation of licensure, and professional association actions for ethical violations.

Professional Guidelines

The APTA's *Guide for Professional Conduct* illustrates ethical principles for therapists relative to documentation practices. Professional conduct standards require that the physical therapist–patient relationship is confidential and cannot be communicated to others without prior written consent from the patient, that peer-reviewed information cannot be released without written permission of the therapist, and that disclosure of medical information without patient consent may be done when necessary to protect the welfare of others in compliance with applicable laws. Physical therapists cannot delegate to less qualified persons activities requiring the skill, knowledge, and judgment of a therapist. Ideally, documentation interpreting health information, examinations, diagnosis, development of the plan of care and goals, identification of precautions and contraindications, reevaluations, discharges, readjustments to plans of care, and follow-up planning are best done when the physical therapist personally records. However, if support staff is used purely to transcribe and the physical therapist signs and/or countersigns such notes, it may be legally sufficient. Ethically, the code specifies that the supervising therapist perform "identification and documentation of precautions, special problems, contraindications, goals, anticipated progress, and plans for reevaluation."[23]

Summary

Healthcare practitioners will be held accountable for knowing, comprehending, and applying relevant state and federal laws and regulations to their specific practice settings. As pertinent laws and regulations are constantly evolving and changing, a practitioner has a professional responsibility to continually update their knowledge. Documentation that is appropriate, complete, and accurate not only contributes to quality patient care but assists with defense against malpractice actions. Medical records containing inappropriate, incomplete, and inaccurate information may result in verdicts against the healthcare organization and provider.

Chapter 7 Review Questions

1. What is informed consent? Explain the relevance to PT documentation.

2. What is HIPAA? What is the relevance to medical records keeping and PT documentation?

3. During what stage of litigation are medical records used? What are they used for?

4. While documentation cannot solve the dilemma of extending treatment for those who have been terminated by third-party payers, what role can it play in premature discharge?

5. What is authentication in documentation?

6. What is the "rule" for the use of abbreviations in documentation? What are the risks and benefits?

7. Explain how errors in documentation should be corrected. What is the role of an addendum?

8. What is counter- or co-signature? In what circumstances is it applicable in PT documentation?

9. What are the benefits of dating and putting the time of treatment on an entry?

10. Are patients/clients entitled to copies of their records? Explain your answer.

Reference

Johns, M., *Health Information Management Technology: An applied approach.* AHIMA, 2002. ISBN 1-58426-056-4.

8

MDS Purpose and Components

The Minimum Data Set (MDS) is a comprehensive assessment instrument designed to describe the medical condition, functional capacity, and treatment regimen of all persons residing in nursing homes in the United States for more than 14 days. The MDS and its companion documentation, the Resident Assessment Instrument (RAI), are mandated by the Social Security Act for all persons receiving Medicare and Medicaid funding. Regulations were amended in the Omnibus Budget Reconciliation Act (OBRA) in 1987 to include all nursing home residents. The form of the MDS in use in fall 2002 is Version 2.0, which was instituted in September of 2000.

The MDS is used as a component of two separate processes. One process is the designation of prospective payment rates received by facilities for the care of each patient. The other is to provide assessment and reassessment data to be used in the Resident Assessment Instrument process that was also mandated by OBRA. Finally, MDS data is utilized by state and local agencies to monitor the quality and safety of skilled nursing facilities. This section will outline the personnel involved, time frames for reporting, and the various applications of MDS/RAI data.

Personnel Reporting on the MDS

Federal law mandates that a Registered Nurse be designated for the coordination of MDS data collection and submission. By law, nurses may document all items of the MDS. Physicians, speech–language pathologists, occupational therapists, activities professionals, dietitians, and physical therapists may also complete MDS items. Information provided by all of the team members described above, along with the patient, the family, direct care providers, such as nursing assistants, and ancillary service personnel may be used in the assessment process. Section AA 9 contains a record of all of the persons completing a portion of the MDS and the specific sections they documented. Signing this section denotes legal responsibility for the accuracy of the information documented in the sections that are signed for.

MDS and the Prospective Payment System

Prior to 1998, nursing homes were reimbursed on a cost basis. Reimbursement was based on the cost of the care provided with no consideration for the amount or type of services a resident actually received. This retrospective approach to reimbursement resulted in a more than 300% increase in healthcare expenditures by Medicare in the early- to mid-1990s. Since 1998, skilled nursing facilities have been paid a prospective, per-diem rate that is based on the care that a patient has received in the recent past and the care that the facility can predict they will need in the near future. Actual cost of the services provided to a patient is not a factor in the reimbursement that a facility receives.

Data collected using the MDS are used to place residents into one of 44 Resource Utilization Groups (RUGs). Each RUG is associated with a corresponding per-diem rate that is further adjusted for regional wage patterns.

Resource Utilization Groups

The 44 RUG categories are divided into seven broad categories that are summarized in Table 8.1. The seven categories are arranged hierarchically by cost with the Rehabilitation category being the most costly. Patients are placed into the Rehabilitation category based on the number of days and minutes of therapy they receive during an assessment period. The next 5 categories are determined by diagnostic criteria and nursing interventions that a patient receives. Time and frequency require-

Table 8.1 RESOURCE UTILIZATION GROUPS (RUGS)

Category	Qualifying Conditions	Stratified By
Rehabilitation Ultra High Very High High Medium Low	Rehabilitation Days and Minutes	ADL Index
Extensive Care	IV Medications Tracheostomy/Extensive Suctioning Parental Nutrition	ADL Index
Special Care	Aphasia Cerebral Palsy Respiratory Infection Multiple Sclerosis Quadriplegia Vomiting with Weight Loss and Fever Dehydration with Fever Surgical Wounds Pressure Ulcers (more than 2 or single Stage 3 or 4) Clinically Complex Comatose Depression/ADL Insulin Dependent Diabetes Hemiplegia Pneumonia Septicemia Dehydration Internal Bleeding	ADL Index
Cognitive Loss	Cognitive Performance Scale	ADL/Nursing Rehab
Behavior Problems		ADL/Nursing Rehab
Decreased Physical Function		ADL/Nursing Rehab

ments for the various rehabilitation RUGs are summarized in Table 8.2. The process of determining a patient's eligibility for placement into the Rehabilitation Category, and their assignment to a specific Rehabilitation RUG is summarized in the next three sections. Two case studies applying the concepts discussed are presented at the end of the chapter.

The rehabilitation category and the next two RUG categories qualify as skilled care under Medicare guidelines. Rehabilitation clinicians should be familiar with the requirements for these categories because a patient must be receiving skilled care to receive Medicare A reimbursement. If a patient qualifies for skilled care based on rehabilitation needs only, the patient and/or their family must be informed immediately at, or prior to, discharge from care or when there is a reduction in therapy because Medicare A benefits may cease and alternate payment methods must be arranged.

ADL Index Score

Section G1 of the MDS is used to generate a composite score, called the ADL (Activities of Daily Living) index, which describes a patient's ability to care for oneself and/or participate in one's care. Activities included in the ADL index are transfers, bed mobility, toileting, and eating. This score is used to assign patients to a sub-group within their RUG category. Patients with higher ADL index scores are more dependent; therefore, it is assumed that increasingly expensive care will be delivered to them. Table 8.3 describes the system for determining ADL index scores from section G1 data.

It is important to consider that the MDS describes a patient's performance in their ADL across seven 24-hour periods and not a patient's best or potential for performance during an observation period. With this in mind, a rehabilitation professional's input should only be one component of the information used to determine the score for an ADL item. A patient's performance with all three shifts of nurses and nursing assistants must be considered and a representative score determined.

Assistance level descriptions differ from those used by most physical and occupational therapists. The ADL index is derived from a combination of two ratings for each activity. The first is a rating for patient performance, which is scored as follows:

0	Independent	Patient received help or oversight on no more than two occasions.
1	Supervision	Patient received help, oversight or cueing 3 or more times and physical assistance no more than 2 times.
2	Limited Assistance	Patient highly involved in activity but requires limb maneuvering assistance 3 or more times and extensive assistance less than two times.
3	Extensive Assistance	Patient performed part of the task but required weight bearing support or total assistance during the last seven days.
4	Total Dependence	Patient did not perform any part of the task.
8	Activity Did Not Occur	

The "Activity Did Not Occur" rating should be used if an activity was not performed during the assessment period for reasons other than patient participation. An example of such a situation would be a patient that did not dress during an assessment period because of a sacral wound care regimen.

ADL support required describes the amount of staff assistance necessary for the patient to accomplish an activity. Items are scored as follows.

0. No setup or staff assistance
1. Set up only
2. One person assistance
3. Two or more person assistance
8. Activity did not occur

Table 8.2
TIME AND FREQUENCY REQUIREMENTS FOR RUGS

RUG Category	Therapy Minutes	Number of Therapies	Therapy Frequency	Actual Rehab Minutes	Estimated Rehab Minutes	Projected Rehab Days	Nursing Rehab
Ultra High	720	2 or more	At least 5 days	NA	NA	NA	NA
Very High	500	One or more	At least 5 days	NA	NA	NA	NA
High	325	One or more	At least 5 days	65	520	8	NA
Medium	150	One or more	At least 5 days	0	240	8	NA
Low	45	One or more	At least 3 days	0	75	5	At least two

Table 8.3
ACTIVITIES OF
DAILY LIVING
INDEX SCORES

Category	Self Performance Score	Staff Support Score	ADL Score
Transfer	4	3 or 8	5
	4	0 to 2	4
	3	3 or 8	5
	3	0 to 2	4
	2	0 to 8	3
	1	0 to 8	1
	0	0 to 8	1
Bed Mobility	4	3 or 8	5
	4	0 to 2	4
	3	3 or 8	5
	3	0 to 2	4
	2	0 to 8	3
	1	0 to 8	1
	0	0 to 8	1
Toilet Use	4	3 or 8	5
	4	0 to 2	4
	3	3 or 8	5
	3	0 to 2	4
	2	0 to 8	3
	1	0 to 8	1
	0	0 to 8	1
Eating	8	0 to 8	3
	4	0 to 8	3
	3	0 to 8	3
	2	0 to 8	2
	1	0 to 8	1
	0	0 to 8	1

Assessment Reference Dates (ARD) Most of the observations on an MDS assessment describe a patient's condition over a 7-day period. Since various members of the interdisciplinary team may be completing the MDS at different times, the MDS coordinator must designate an assessment reference date. The assessment reference date is the final 24-hour period of the 7-day MDS observation interval. Because of this all MDS documentation should be dated after the ARD.

Grace Days The MDS/PPS system allows for a certain degree of flexibility in the determination of assessment reference dates. Each of the MDS time frames described above has a range of possible ARD. All MDS may have an ARD before the assessment designated date (for example the 30-day MDS may have an ARD as early as day 23).

The days beyond the designated day of an MDS assessment are called grace days. These dates are built into the system so that a facility can assess days that are truly representative of a patient's condition and treatment. Grace days can be used to accommodate decreased participation in care and therapy, associated with adjustment to a new facility and acuity of illness. Time away from the facility for tests, doctor visits, brief hospitalizations, and family visitation are accommodated for established patients as well. The grace day system also allows facilities to capture a representative number of therapy days and minutes for patients admitted late in the day or week.

Special Treatments, Procedures, and Programs

MDS section P Item 1B a through c records the number of days and minutes that the patient receives physical, occupational, speech, respiratory, and psychological therapy during the 7-day observation period. This record of the rehabilitation services that the patient received is used to determine the patient's eligibility for placement in a Rehabilitation RUG for all MDS assessments except the 5-day MDS.

For physical therapy minutes to qualify for inclusion on the MDS several criteria must be met.

1. Treatments must be based on an active treatment plan that was generated by a physical therapy evaluation performed on the patient as a resident of the skilled nursing facility. A PT evaluation performed in the acute care hospital is not sufficient to initiate a course of treatment in a nursing home.

2. Treatments must be ordered by a physician.

3. All treatment minutes must be performed by a physical therapist but may include the assistance of a physical therapy student, aide, or volunteer.

OR

Treatments must be performed by a physical therapy assistant under the supervision of a physical therapist.

4. Therapy provided to patients in groups of four or fewer persons by a PT or PTA may be included in section P if group therapy is less than 25% of the therapy received by a patient during the observation period.

It is critical that the time frame recorded in therapy documentation in the medical record agrees with the minutes and days of therapy entered in this item. In January 2000, the U.S. Office of the Inspector General (OIG) reported that Section P documentation along with ADL Index scores are the two areas of the MDS that have the worst agreement with documentation in the rest of the medical record. The OIG made a point that the facilities inspected did not show a clear trend toward over-reporting therapy minutes, which suggests that facilities are not trying to defraud the Medicare system. As a result of this disagreement the OIG recommended that these areas be scrutinized in further inspections and for revision of the items themselves.

Medicare 5-Day Therapy Supplement

Medicare 5-day assessments must include documentation on MDS section T item 1a and 1c if a physician has ordered PT, OT, or SLP services during the initial assessment period. This section provides an estimation of the amount of therapy a patient will receive during the first 15 days of a skilled nursing facility stay. This section will be used to determine the patient's eligibility for rehabilitation RUGs for the first 15 days of a qualifying Medicare A reimbursed stay.

Predicted days and minutes of therapy are not used for placing patients in the Rehab Very High and Ultra High categories using the 5-day MDS. Actual performance of therapy, recorded on Section P of the 14-day MDS is used to qualify for these RUG categories.

The procedure for determining estimated therapy days is as follows:

1. Count the days that a patient received at least one qualifying, 15 minute long, therapy treatment through the ARD to determine actual therapy days.

2. Use therapy orders, treatment plans, and the policies of the facility to project the number of days the patient should receive at least one qualifying therapy treat-

ment, starting the day after the ARD, through day 14 to determine the number of predicted therapy days.

3. Actual Therapy Days + Predicted Therapy Days = Estimated Therapy Days

The procedure for determining estimated number of therapy minutes is as follows:

1. Count the number of qualifying therapy minutes that the patient received through the ARD to determine actual therapy minutes.

2. Use therapy orders, treatment plans, and the policies of the facility to project the number of minutes of therapy the patient should receive, starting the day after the ARD, through day 14 to determine the number of predicted therapy days.

3. Actual Therapy Minutes + Predicted Therapy Minutes = Estimated Therapy Minutes

Walking When Most Self-Sufficient

MDS section T items 2a through 2e describe the patient's best ambulation/gait performance. This is the only section on the MDS rating best performance as opposed to usual or representative performance. Physical therapy or nursing staff can complete this item if the following criteria are met:

1. ADL self performance score for transfers is 0, 1, 2, 3.

2. The resident receiving physical therapy for gait training or physical therapy for gait training has been discharged in the past six months.

Physical therapy or nursing rehabilitation notes should support the score recorded in this item in terms of distance, time assistance device, and the amount of staff assistance received.

Resident Assessment Instrument Process

The MDS is used for an important set of processes beyond the MDS/PPS system. The MDS is a data collection tool designed to cue facilities to develop care plans that will impact critical components of a resident's health and quality of life. MDS data are also used to assist state agencies in monitoring the quality and safety of skilled nursing facilities.

Resident Assessment Protocols and Care Planning Scores on specific items in the MDS "trigger" a Resident Assessment Protocol (RAP) for a given area. The trigger legend is a component of many printed versions of the MDS that indicate that an MDS item score identifies an area requiring further assessment by the interdisciplinary team. For example, a patient will trigger a RAP for pressure ulcers if they are scored as being incontinent of bowel, dependent in bed mobility, having diminished sensation, or being essentially bed-bound. There are 18 RAP areas, which are summarized in Table 8.4. RAP areas that will commonly involve evaluation and subsequent care planning by physical therapists include physical restraints, falls, decreased ADL, and pressure ulcers.

Discipline-specific documentation along with patient history and diagnostic testing information will be used to make decisions on the course of action necessary to address a given RAP area. If any of this documentation indicates the need for interdisciplinary intervention, a written care plan must be generated. All initial and annual MDS/RAI assessments must contain a RAP summary, which contains a summary of the information described above and the rationale involved in the decisions made. The MDS coordinator generates RAP summaries at the completion of the RAI process.

Quality Indicators. The quality control component of the RAI is the Quality Indicator (QI) system. There are MDS items tracking 24 negative outcomes summarized in Table 8.5. This data is used by state agencies to track individual facilities performance against benchmarked quality standards for an area and to identify facilities

Table 8.4
RESIDENT
ASSESSMENT
PROTOCOL (RAP)

1 Delirium	10 Activities
2 Cognitive Loss/Dementia	11 Falls
3 Communication	12 Nutritional Status
4 Communication	13 Feeding Tubes
5 ADL	14 Dehydration/Fluid Status
6 Urinary Incontinence/Indwelling Catheter	15 Dental Care
7 Psycho/Social Well-Being	16 Pressure Ulcers
8 Mood State	17 Psychotropic Drug Use
9 Behavioral Symptoms	18 Physical Restraints

that fall below critical standards. The QI system also facilitates focused inspections by providing inspectors with lists of patients having experienced negative outcomes in the recent past.

Timeframes for MDS and RAI Completion   OBRA requires that a comprehensive admission assessment including the MDS and the entire RAI process be completed by day 14 of a patients stay. This process is completed annually for all nursing home residents. Quarterly MDS re-assessments are also completed for the duration of a patient's stay.

Table 8.5
QUALITY INDICATORS

1 Incidence of new fractures
2 Prevalence of falls
3 Prevalence of behavior problems affecting others
4 Prevalence of symptoms of depression
5 Prevalence of depression without antidepressants
6 Nine plus medications
7 Incidence of cognitive impairments
8 Prevalence of bladder or bowel incontinence
9 Prevalence of bowel and bladder incontinence without pain
10 Prevalence of indwelling catheter
11 Prevalence of fecal impaction
12 Prevalence of UTI
13 Prevalence of weight loss
14 Prevalence of tube feeding
15 Prevalence of dehydration
16 Prevalence of bedfast residents
17 Incidence of decline in late loss ADL
18 Incidence of decrease in ROM
19 Prevalence of antipsychotics in the absence of psychosis
20 Prevalence of anti-anxiety/hypnotics
21 Prevalence of hypnotic use > 2×/week
22 Prevalence of physical restraints
23 Prevalence of little or no activity
24 Prevalence of stage 1 to 4 pressure ulcers

In addition, the Medicare/PPS system also requires that an MDS be completed on day 5 and day 14. With certain restrictions, either of these assessments can be used to fulfill the OBRA admission assessment requirement. MDS assessments are also required for day 30, 60, 90, and 100. The 90-day MDS may fulfill the requirements for the OBRA quarterly re-assessment.

The 5-day MDS is used to determine the patients RUG for the first 14 days of a patient's stay. Each of the subsequent Medicare PPS assessments is used to determine a patient's RUG for the period through the due date for the next assessment. Table 8.6 summarizes the PPS and OBRA reporting schedules.

Significant Change in Status Assessment A new MDS with an RAI must be completed if the facility determines that the patient experiences a significant improvement or decline. A decline should resolve with time or standard medical treatment. The status change should also require the interdisciplinary review of the care plan, affect at least two aspects of the patient's care, and result in assignment to a new RUG category.

Other Medicare Required Assessment (OMRA) An "Other Medicare Required Assessment" (OMRA) must be completed within 8 days after all therapies have been completed for patients that satisfy requirements for another skilled care RUG. This assessment is designed to establish a new prospective payment for the balance of a patient's 100 days of Medicare skilled nursing.

Summary

Use of the MDs in skilled nursing facility setting is challenging. However, it is necessary on an initial and ongoing basis for all SNF patients and residents in order to comply with federal regulations. Although this serves as an introduction to the instrument, clinicians should refer to the MDS 2.0 Users' Manual during their first attempts to negotiate the MDS and RAI system.

Table 8.6
REPORTING SCHEDULE

Type of MDS	Possible ARD	Determines Reimbursement for Days
5 Day MDS PPS and OBRA	Day 1 to 8 Includes 3 grace days	1 to 14
14 Day MDS PPS	Day 11 to 19 Includes 5 grace days	15 to 30
14 Day MDS PPS and OBRA	Day 11 to 14 No grace days if OBRA admission	15 to 30
30 Day MDS	Day 21 to 34 Includes 5 grace days	31 to 60
60 Day MDS	Day 50 to 64 Includes 5 grace days	60 to 90
90 day MDS PPS and OBRA Quarterly	Day 80 to 92 Includes 3 grace days	90 to 100

Chapter 8 Review Cases and Exercises

Case One

Section T. Therapy Supplement   Mr. G. was admitted on Monday, January 14 at 9 A.M. after an acute hospitalization for CHF. He presents with decreased endurance, decreased high-level balance, and mild to moderate dementia. PT and OT evaluations were ordered on admission. After the evaluations, orders were received for PT and OT 3 times per week for 4 weeks. The MDS coordinator designated Friday, January 18 as the ARD for the 5 Day MDS.

To determine the estimated number of therapy days for MDS Section T, item 1c:

1. Mr. G. received at least 15 minutes of therapy on 5 days through the ARD.

2. Mr. G. is scheduled for at least 15 minutes of therapy on 5 additional days through day 14.

3. 5 + 5 = 10 (Actual days + Projected Days = Estimated Days)

To determine the estimated number of therapy minutes for MDS Section T, Item 1d:

4. Mr. G. received 75 minutes of PT treatment and 90 minutes of PT treatment through the ARD.

5. Mr. G. is scheduled to receive 90 additional minutes of PT treatment and 90 additional minutes of OT through day 14.

6. 165 + 180 = 345 (Actual Minutes + Projected Minutes = Estimated Minutes)

Based on the therapy performance and schedule described above, Mr. G qualifies for the Rehab High Category.

ADL Index Score   Mr. G. requires set up for transferring, bed mobility, and eating and requires physical assistance of one person for toileting 4 or 5 times per week.

These levels of assistance qualify Mr. G for an ADL Score of 6, which would place him in the Rehab High A RUG. In an urban area in April 2001, the facility that cared for Mr. G would have received $260.46 per day.

If Mr. G. received the same amount of therapy but was dependent for all tasks, he would qualify for the Rehab High C RUG and the facility caring for him would have received $313.52 per day.

Case Two

Section T. Therapy Supplement   Mrs. S. was admitted for open reduction and internal fixation of a hip fracture on Wednesday, October 7. An OT and PT evaluation was ordered on the day of admission. OT completed its evaluation on Thursday, October 8. Mrs. S. began vomiting in the afternoon and did not receive her PT evaluation. Mrs. S. refused all therapies on October 9 secondary to nausea. The PT evaluation was completed on Monday, October 12.

The MDS coordinator designated Wednesday, October 14 as the ARD using all 3 grace days to accommodate Mrs. S.'s nausea and vomiting

To determine the estimated number of therapy days for MDS Section T, item 1c:

7. Mrs. S. received at least 15 minutes of therapy on 3 days through the ARD.

8. Mrs. S is scheduled for at least 15 minutes of therapy on 7 additional days through day 14.

9. 3 + 7 = 10 (Actual days + Projected Days = Estimated Days)

To determine the estimated number of therapy minutes for MDS Section T, item 1d:

10. Mrs. S. received 90 minutes of PT treatment and 90 minutes of PT treatment through the ARD.

11. Mrs. S. is scheduled to receive 210 additional minutes of PT treatment and 210 additional minutes of OT through day 14.

12. $180 + 420 = 600$ (Actual Minutes + Projected Minutes = Estimated Minutes)

Based on the therapy performance and schedule described above Mrs. S. qualifies at least for the Rehab High Category. Medicare guidelines require patients to actually perform the required minutes and days of therapy for the Rehab High and Very High categories. If Mrs. S. performs all of her scheduled therapy days she will qualify for the Rehab Very High Category.

9

Medicare and Non-Medicare Content Principles

According to the APTA *Guide to Physical Therapist Practice,* there are 25 categories of tests and measures in physical therapy (PT): aerobic capacity, anthropometric characteristics, arousal/attention and cognition, assistive and adaptive devices, circulation (arterial, venous, lymphatic), cranial and peripheral nerve integrity, environmental/home and work (job, school, play) barriers, ergonomics and body mechanics, gait/locomotion and balance, integument integrity, joint integrity and mobility, motor function (motor control and learning), muscle performance (strength, power, endurance), neuromotor development and sensory integration, orthotic/protective and supportive devices, pain, posture, prosthetic requirements, range of motion (including muscle length), reflex integrity, self-care and home management (activities of daily living [ADL] and instrumental activities of daily living [IADL]), sensory integrity, ventilation and respiration/gas exchange, and work (job/school/play), and community and leisure integration or reintegration.

The therapist selects those tests and measures most appropriate to the patient/client's signs, symptoms, and concerns using the clinical decision-making model.

For Medicare purposes, tests and measures should be focused on activities related to necessary function versus leisure, and those impairments directly impacting that necessary or essential function. Essential function includes: adequate aerobic endurance to perform activities such as transitional movements and transfers, bed mobility, gait on a variety of surfaces or if non-ambulatory or limited in gait, other locomotion (i.e., wheelchair, power-operated vehicle, or power wheelchair), negotiating doorways and different surfaces, avoidance of objects, safety, balance in standing and ADL. In some instances, tests and measures include IADL and negotiating public transportation if a beneficiary is still working, or receiving treatment on an outpatient basis. Pain, in the absence of dysfunction, is not a qualifier for skilled physical therapy. However, if the patient/client is reporting pain and it effects functions not necessarily apparent or measurable in the clinic, close attention must be paid to patient/client monitoring of improvement external to the clinic as a measure of success. Examples of this are sleeping through the night or if driving is necessary (even if it is to and from medical appointments), the ability to safely turn the head, sit for a prescribed length of time, and operate the vehicle safely. Lack of sleep can result in impairment in judgment and fatigue, endurance limitations, depression, and weakness. Specific cardiac rehabilitation is not considered a skilled Medicare-approved PT procedure, although respiratory programs may be in certain circumstances. Individuals with cardiac problems qualify for skilled PT secondary to weakness, functional decline, gait abnormalities, etc.

In the non-Medicare adult context, the concept of function may be more generic in scope, encompassing leisure and lifestyle. However, as in Medicare, pain in the absence of functional limitation will most likely not be reimbursable unless the patient/client has been specifically referred for pain management or a pain program, and it has been pre-approved by the payer. There may be limited reimbursement to instruct an individual in techniques that may help manage the pain and facilitate function depending on the payer source.

Wellness programs are not reimbursed as skilled physical therapy in Medicare or non-Medicare venues. Specific cardiac and respiratory intervention may be covered in non-Medicare venues depending on the payer.

Medicare: Inpatient and Outpatient

Skilled Content Recommendations: CMS 700

If the PT facility is not billing Medicare or is billing using the CMS 1500, the same content is required in the documentation. The data entered on the CMS 1500 does not include status or problems, but rather diagnostic and corresponding CPT codes.

AUTHOR'S NOTE

Content categories are relevant for all initial examinations and content as appropriate to non-Medicare evaluations (the shorter the form, the easier to find information). The 700 contains content for justifying care. It is not the actual bill.

The CMS 1500 form is a single page (see Appendix B) with boxes for patient identifiers, provider identifiers, onset date, start of care date (SOC), primary medical diagnosis, treatment diagnosis, visits from SOC, type of service, physician, and PT information. The CMS 1500 also contains blocks of blank space for plan of treatment functional goals (short and long term in weeks, not to exceed four), plan frequency and duration, certification dates, prior hospitalization (as applicable), initial assessment (history, medical complications, level of function at start of care, and reason for referral), and functional level (at end of billing period). There are also progress report boxes to indicate whether to continue service or discharge (DC). In order to ensure appropriate completion, PTs should add written categories to the form. If entered in small enough font, adequate space is available if PTs enter only what is necessary.

EXAMPLE

Sample Plan Checklist:

___ Therapeutic exercise for UE/LE/Trunk: progressive strengthening/ROM/ endurance

___ Neuromuscular reeducation: balance training, proprioceptive training, coordination training (This category may be challenged by Medicare PTs.)

___ Therapeutic activities: transfer training, functional training, bed mobility

___ Gait training

___ Wheelchair training

___ Patient/caregiver education/training

___ Safety training

___ (Fill in others as indicated based on CPT codes)

___ Other

Initial Assessment (Fill in Blanks)

History of Current Illness

Past medical history _____

Prior level of function (prior to current episode) _____

Reason for referral (should be functionally oriented and may match treatment diagnosis if functional) _____

Cognition (alert, oriented to person, place, time) _____

Follows _____ step directions:
    Verbal/gesture/combination _____
    Safety awareness _____
    Precautions _____
    Endurance: respiratory/cardiac_____
    Balance: Sitting: Static _____ Dynamic____
                 Standing: Static _____ Dynamic_____
Other categories
    Strength: 0/5 to 5/5 scale _____
    Other muscle performance _____
    ROM (expressed as fraction out of "normal ranges") _____
    Tone: low, high, rigidity, spasticity (e.g., Modified Ashworth Scale)_____
    Pain: location/grade 0/10 to 10/10, activity affected_____
    Skin integrity_____
    Sensation: light touch, pain, proprioception _____
    Bed mobility _____
    Rolling: L/R _____
    Supine <> sit: log sit and short sit _____
    Scooting: side to side, up and down _____
    Transfers: Sit <> stand_____
Stand pivot
    W/C, chair <> bed/mat_____
    Gait: device, pattern, dependence _____
    WC management: manual, electric wheelchair, or vehicle_____
    Balance _____
    Posture _____
    Other _____
Rehabilitation potential (relative to PT) _____
    Plan of treatment functional goals _____
_____
_____

Since all information using this format is on a single page, it is not necessary to write a separate problem and summary. Reason for referral should include this information. However, each category with a deficit noted should have a corresponding short-term and long-term goal as indicated. Impairment-based goals should be included but linked to the functional end.

EXAMPLES

Medical diagnosis: Contusions left hip (hematoma), low back pain

PT diagnosis: gait abnormality, contusions, low back pain, weakness

Reason for referral: Dependent for gait, transfers, weakness

BLEs and back pain, dependence for ADL, IADL since she fell

Prior level of function: Lived alone in first floor apartment, I in all ADL & IADL, drives own car

Strength: LE: 3+/5 proximal, 3/5 distal, UE: 4-/5 gross strength

AROM: shoulders: 0° to 160/180° of flex/abd, fingers maintained in minimal flexion with arthritic changes noted

The categories indicated above may be adjusted depending on the type of clientele a facility sees. Remember that the treatment diagnosis must be consistent with the planned interventions, the deficits identified, and the short- and long-term goals. All categories indicated correspond to the categories in the APTA *Guide to Physical Therapist Practice.*

Patient/Client Goals: Medicare and Non-Medicare

According to the *Guide to Physical Therapist Practice,* goals and expected outcomes are categorized together. Following are the categories of goals (based on increases or improvement) with summaries of the skills that should be considered when writing patient/client goals. Please note that although categories may be stated in broad, general terms, they must be stated specifically in the actual plan for an individual patient/client. These are applicable across all settings and are applicable to patients/clients through the lifespan.

Impact of Pathology/ Pathophysiology

The impact of the pathology or pathophysiology is the reason the patient/client needs PT. This is the PT diagnosis, PT problems, the relationship between the medical problem and/or the resulting functional deficits. Patient pathology may include reduction of edema or lymphedema, reduction of joint inflammation and swelling, reduction in soft tissue swelling or tone, enhanced wound healing, or tissue restriction reduction.

Impact on Impairments

The impact of PT on the patient's impairment can take on several different forms. Among the changes one might see as a result of PT are: increased endurance and aerobic capacity; decreased energy expenditure; increased ROM; improved muscle performance (strength, power, endurance); decreased breathing effort; changes in motor control (synergy, patterns, coordination); improved balance; increased postural control; improved integument and joint integrity; increased sensory awareness; improved gait and locomotion; increased weight bearing; optimal joint alignment and use (i.e., prosthesis, orthosis); optimal loading on a body part; and enhanced tissue perfusion and oxygenation.

Impact on Functional Limitations

PT's impact on the patient's functional limitation includes decreased levels of dependence or need for assistance, improved ability to perform tasks, increased tolerance to positional changes, and increased performance of and independence in ADL and IADL with or without devices. (In the *Guide to Physical Therapist Practice* model, gait-related activities are listed under impairments.)

Impact on Disabilities

As the patient continues PT, his or her disabilities will be impacted in several ways. The patient's ability to resume performance of life roles, such as returning to work or school, returning home (if PT was inpatient), and resuming those leisure activities once challenging or impossible due to the impairment.

Risk Reduction/ Prevention

During and after PT, the patient should experience a reduction in risk factors such as surgical precautions and weight bearing. The patient will also experience an awareness of surroundings, compensation for sensory or vision loss, awareness of potential for skin breakdown, appropriate awareness of abilities versus inabilities, decreased risk of developing secondary problems, protection of body parts is achieved, pressure on tissues is reduced, and increased understanding of assistive devices and their use as well as safety awareness.

Impact on Health, Wellness, and Fitness

As the PT continues, the patient will gradually experience improved health status and increased overall wellness. Physical function and capacity are improved, allowing the patient to improve physical fitness and activity.

Patient/Client Satisfaction

Although there are multiple factors to consider regarding patient satisfaction, the most relevant to intervention goals are improved sense of well-being and decreased stressors. The patient's satisfaction is based mainly on the level and timeliness of goal achievement (see Tables 9.1, 9.2, and 9.3 for sample patient goals).

Table 9.1
SAMPLE PATIENT
GOALS

Deficit/Finding/Problem	Short-Term Goal 2 Weeks (include date)
Endurance poor (based on scale)	Increase to poor + to eliminate constant respiratory symptoms and fatigue at rest
Static sitting 3+/5	Increase to 4–/5 to reduce fall risk in sitting associated with COG changes
Dynamic sitting 3+/5	Increase to 4/5 to prevent falls associated with COG changes, reaching and bending in sit
Static standing 3/5	Increase to 4/5 to minimize fall risk in standing activities
Dynamic standing 2+/5 with rolling walker	Increase to 3/5 to begin decreasing fall risk on indoor surfaces
Rolling L/R modified with bedrails, limited assist 10% for lower trunk	Progress to limited assist 5% without rails to facilitate change of position for skin protection and to facilitate sleep through the night
Supine <> sit limited assist 25%	Supine <> sit limited assist 10%
Scooting limited assist 25%	Scooting limited assist 10%
Transfers: sit <> stand limited assist 25%	Transfers: sit <> stand limited assist 10%
WC <> bed/mat limited assist 25%	WC <> bed/mat with supervision
ROM: within functional limits with exception of B ankles: 0 from neutral	With verbal cues, will perform exercises to be performed in room and at home to increase ankle ROM and facilitate performance of functional activities
	10° of Active Assisted dorsiflexion
Strength within grossly 3+/5 to 4–/5, with limited endurance to sustain activities	Strength consistent in 4–/5 range in order to sustain movement during functional activities such as gait, standing
Gait front wheeled rolling walker step to, ↓ knee flexion L with swing, ↓ initial contact L/R, ↓ cadence, forward flexed trunk, limited assist 25%	Gait with rolling walker level surfaces 50′ to 80′ to allow gait to bathroom and dining
WC management dependent	IWC management on level and carpeted surfaces to allow safe locomotion and promote I mobility in the short term

Table 9.2 SAMPLE PATIENT GOALS	2 Weeks: (should include actual date, not # weeks)
	1. Contact guard: Gait with standard walker on even (or level) surfaces, WBAT, 50′, with ability to make 180° turn and step backward without toe drag, with single rest of one minute, at half normal speed: ~ 40 meters/minute
	2. Ability to open and close doors with handles with Limited Assistance: 25%, while using walker
	3. Supervision and verbal cues for transfers sit <> stand
	4. Supervision and verbal cues for stand pivot transfer bed <> chair
	5. R dorsiflexion strength of 3+/5 (from 3–/5) with elimination of toe drag to enable safe gait
	6. Improve standing balance from _____ to _____ without walker to prevent falls when standing for activities that preclude holding walker; i.e., dressing, hygiene, kitchen related
	7. Increase endurance for functional activity from _____ to _____
	8. Improve wheelchair mobility on even surface with ability to lock and unlock brakes, flip foot rests and leg rests, and negotiate doorways
	9. Pt will demonstrate ability to perform exercises in room
	3 Weeks: (should include actual date, not # weeks)
	1. Improve gait with standard walker on even and uneven (rugs, concrete, grass) surfaces, with ability to execute turns spontaneously all directions with heel/toe pattern 100′ without rest at normal speed of 82 m/minute
	2. Improve ability to negotiate doors (open and close) without loss of balance
	3. Improve transfers sit <> stand
	4. Improve stand pivot transfers bed <> chair, toilet, shower
	5. Increase R dorsiflexion strength from 3–/5 to 4–/5 to eliminate toe drag/drop foot for sustained safe gait up to 100′
	6. Improve standing balance from _____ to _____ for safe, stable standing for self-care activities, bathroom and kitchen tasks
	7. Improve wheelchair mobility on even and uneven surfaces (rugs, concrete, grass) for longer, functional distances
	8. Pt will demonstrate ability to perform home exercises independently

Table 9.3 SAMPLE PATIENT PROBLEMS AND GOALS	68 y.o. male hospitalized 5 days
	Medical Diagnosis: resolving left lower lobe atelectasis, HTN, pneumonia
	PT diagnosis: gait disturbance, weakness
	Prior level of function: multiple falls over 6 months, lives with daughter in single-story house, ambulatory with standard walker
	Precautions: cardiac, falls, universal
	Alert, oriented to person, place, time
	Able to follow single step instructions
	Vision: R cataract
	Hard of hearing
	Safety awareness: poor
	Skin intact, no edema noted
	At rest: Vital signs: BP: 135/85 R: 24, shallow, Pulse: 90

**Table 9.3
(Continued)**

Deficit/finding/problem	Short term goal 2 weeks (include date)
Endurance poor (based on scale)	Increase to poor + to eliminate constant respiratory symptoms and fatigue at rest
Static sitting 3+/5	Increase to 4-/5 to reduce fall risk in sitting associated with COG changes
Dynamic sitting 3+/5	Increase to 4/5 to prevent falls associated with COG changes, reaching and bending in sit
Static standing 3/5	Increase to 4/5 to minimize fall risk in standing activities
Dynamic standing with rolling walker 2+/5	Increase to 3/5 to begin decreasing fall risk on indoor surfaces
Rolling L/R modified with bedrails, limited assist 10% for lower trunk	Progress to limited assist 5% without rails to facilitate change of position for skin protection and to facilitate sleep through the night
Supine <> sit limited assist 25%	Supine <> sit limited assist 10%
Scooting limited assist 25%	Scooting limited assist 10%
Transfers: sit<> stand limited assist 25%	Transfers: sit<> stand limited assist 10%
WC <> bed/mat limited assist 25%	WC <> bed/mat with supervision
ROM: within functional limits with exception of B ankles: 0 from neutral	With verbal cues, will perform exercises to be performed in room and at home to increase ankle ROM and facilitate performance of functional activities 10 of Active Assisted dorsiflexion
Strength within grossly 3+/5 to 4-/5, with limited endurance to sustain activities	Strength consistent in 4-/5 range in order to sustain movement during functional activities such as gait, standing
Gait front wheeled rolling walker step to, ↓ knee flexion L with swing, ↓ initial contact L/R, ↓ cadence, forward flexed trunk, limited assist 25%	Gait with rolling walker level surfaces 50 to 80' to allow gait to bathroom and dining
WC management dependent	I WC management on level and carpeted surfaces to allow safe locomotion and promote I mobility in the short term

Plan of Treatment with Functional Goals

Since all patient goal information is on a single page on a 700 series form or similar self-designed form, it is not necessary to write a separate problem summary. The reason for referral should include this information. However, each category with a deficit noted should have a corresponding short- and long-term goal as indicated. Impairment-based goals should be included but linked to the functional end. The following examples lists several functionally oriented goals in PT.

EXAMPLE

Functionally Oriented Goals

- Pain reduction from 8/10 to 1/10 during prolonged sitting for up to one hour, to allow resumption of work at computer station, with 10-minute break at end of hour

- Resolution of disk protrusion with resultant resolution of right shifted standing posture to allow unguarded, pain free gait in order to resume ADL and IADL activities, leisure, work, family responsibilities

- Restore full, stable cervical rotation to allow safe independent driving: checking mirrors, backing up, in order to return to drive to work, etc.

- Increase UE elevation to 160° bilaterally to allow independent dressing including overhead garments, self-care activities, over head reaching activities in kitchen, adjust auto mirrors

---

Intervention—Plan

The categories used in the Intervention—Plan include therapeutic exercise for Cervical area/Trunk, such as progressive strengthening, ROM, endurance, and stabilization; neuromuscular therapy, such as proprioceptive and coordination training; manipulation and mobilization; and therapeutic massage. These categories may be adjusted depending on the type of clientele a facility sees. Remember that the treatment diagnosis must be consistent with the planned interventions, the deficits identified and the short- and long-term goals. All categories indicated correspond to the categories in the *Guide to Physical Therapist Practice* (see Table 9.4 for a sample intervention—plan).

Content: Continuation of Care

Words and Phrases to Assist with Content

Remember that the documentation includes baseline or initial examination data, anticipated goals based on the identified patient/client problems, and the interim progress described relative to the baseline and goal. All deficits must ultimately be linked to the function they impact.

Table 9.4
SAMPLE
INTERVENTION—
PLAN

Therapeutic exercise for UE/LE/Trunk: progressive strengthening/ROM/endurance
Neuromuscular: reeducation: balance training, proprioceptive training, coordination training
Therapeutic activities: transfer training, functional training
Gait training
Wheelchair training
Bed mobility training
Patient/caregiver education/training
Safety training
Other _____

Anthropometric Anthropometric measurement is used in PT to describe overall height, weight, body mass index, as well as overall body type, extremity or extremity segment size, and how size relates to function. The therapist should describe fat distribution as applicable, presence of obesity, and weight control problems. Measurements must be objective. If a scale is not available, record observations and ask the patient/client height and weight.

Joint Integrity and Mobility Joint integrity and mobility in PT is expressed in terms of joint play and range of motion (ROM) and should be listed as a fraction of the measured and full range. These measurements should be taken at baseline, throughout care, and at discharge using the appropriate goniometer. If the measurements are visually estimated, be sure to indicate this in the record.

EXAMPLE

Shoulder flexion: AROM: 80°/180°, PROM 120°/180°

Deviations: from joint and body planes, with excursions in distances

EXAMPLE

15° L genu valgum

5 inches of spinal excursion in forward flexion

Joint Motion: quality of motion, i.e., end feel, painful arc, bony block, capsular patterns, glide, laxity, or restriction

EXAMPLE

Provocation responses/tests: + anterior drawer sign L knee

Patient description/reports of pain (objectively measure) or other during activities and movement

EXAMPLE

Patient CO (complains of) grinding in shoulders with elevation and functional use

Patient CO clicking in L knee during walking and cycling

Muscle Performance Strength and muscle performance should always be expressed as a fraction. These measurements should be taken at baseline, progressively throughout care and at termination of care, based on a pre-determined scale of 0/5 to 5/5 or scale of preference. Avoid verbiage only in correspondence regarding muscle performance because it is often misunderstood and considered better than it is.

EXAMPLE

R quads 3/5 at initial examination

Goal: Increase R quad to 4/5 to enable safe standing without device as required for job

Interim statement of progress: Pt's R quad strength has increased from 3/5 to 3+/5 decreasing frequency of buckling with weight transfer on and off limb in standing

Passive tension, length measurement with patient/client CO pain, pulling, or tenderness during multisegmental movement

---

EXAMPLE

Active R SLR: 70°

In long sit: fingertip to toes with knees straight = 3 inches with CO pulling in low back musculature and hamstrings resulting in inability to don stockings

Soft tissue density, turgor, response to movement

EXAMPLE

In standing, left trunk side bending limited secondary to R quadratus lumborum spasm

R quadratus lumborum tender to palpation

Trigger point or tender point location and radiation patterns as applicable, using finger pressure or a pressure meter designed for assessment

---

EXAMPLE

Trigger point L upper trapezius with radiation into shoulder with moderate pressure, limiting ability to position head to read or turn during driving

Muscle Contraction quality: smooth versus interrupted, tremulous or rigid or otherwise

---

EXAMPLE

Unable to sustain smooth muscle contraction to oppose

R thumb to R forefinger, assists with L hand

Unable to sustain smooth muscle contraction to control hand during attempts to write or use keyboard without error

Sustained muscle endurance to perform movement with multiple repetitions or sustained contraction

---

Neuromotor Development and Sensory Integration Neuromotor development and sensory integration is developed over time in PT. Neuromotor skills are developed by gradually performing muscle stretch reflexes and deep tendon reflexes (DTRs).

EXAMPLE

R biceps = 2+ (normal)

L patella = 1 (hyporeflexive)

Electrical assessment over time: EMG, nerve conduction, etc.

Synergic dominance and tone, abnormal reflexes and ability to initiate and isolate movement in relation to gravity and body position

---

EXAMPLE

Unable to isolate elbow flexion and extension on table top for support, interfering with eating, writing, self-care

Modified Ashworth Scale:

5/5: Normal tone: no increase or decrease

4/5: Slight tone increase, catch and release, or minimal resistance at end of range

> 3/5: Slight increase in tone manifested by catch, followed by minimal resistance
>
> 2/5: More marked tone through most of the range of motion but affected part(s) easily moved
>
> 1/5: Considerable increase in muscle tone, passive movement is difficult
>
> 0/5: Affected part(s) rigid in flexion or extension

Sensation impairment: distributions affected and specific sensation

---

AUTHOR'S NOTE

Although the Modified Ashworth includes fractions from 0/5 to 5/5, the numbers alone should be avoided since they may be confused for strength.

EXAMPLE

Sensation absent in L5 dermatome, resulting in potential for injury, skin breakdown

Sensory integration with environment: state of system

EXAMPLE

Demonstrates tactile defensiveness to all external stimuli including clothing and touch

Demonstrates increase in observable synergies in response to noise in room, interfering with ability to isolate movement and preventing functional use of extremities

Developmental reflex impact on movement patterns and posturing

EXAMPLE

R ATNR dominance preventing neutral supine positioning, unable to roll right or left preventing rolling.

Developmental level: described in terms of milestones usually indicated on standardized forms for standardized assessment.

Motor Function, Motor Control, and Learning When evaluating motor function, motor control, and learning, the PT should observe movement patterns, postural control, and unprovoked movement.

EXAMPLE

Demonstrates severe kyphosis in sitting, limiting UE elevation and diaphragm excursion associated with increased respiratory rate and accessory muscle use.

Time to complete tasks: slowness when it interferes with function is justification of care especially in task that need immediate response such as toileting.

EXAMPLE

Patient transferred wheelchair to bed with minimal assist or limited assist of 25% in 5 minutes, stand/pivot to R.

Sequencing and cuing for task accomplishment.

EXAMPLE

Requires 1 step instructions with tactile cues to execute sit to partial stand

Recall/repeat ability to perform a task in a different context or at a different time.

EXAMPLE

Now able to perform stand pivot transfer from WC to Mat table with supervision. As yet, requires moderate or extensive assist at 50% from WC to bed at same height.

Response to therapeutic exercise intervention such as rhythmic stabilization and contract-relax.

EXAMPLE

Able to maintain erect trunk posture in response and maintain for 2 minutes with verbal cues.

Coma level description using standardized scales such as the Glasgow or Rancho Los Amigos.

Coordination Skills

Balance.   The therapist should describe balance and/or record balance ratings on standardized scales or from computerized equipment. Always use functional terms rather than good, fair, or poor, which are not objective, measurable terms. There are standard instruments such as the Berg Balance and Timed Get Up and Go and Functional Reach, which assist in qualifying and quantifying balance. One can also use a 0/5 to 5/5 scale for describing balance in sit and stand, static and dynamic.

EXAMPLE

Maintains vertical position in standing for 60 seconds without cues or support. Self-corrects to vertical 50% of time with verbal cues. Requires bilateral UE support to maintain balance during gait. Resting posture is 15° to right of vertical. Falls to left 3 out of 5 times when perturbed from right. Consistently able to reach beyond base of support without falling. Falls to left when changing direction of gait 80% of time and relies on constant cues to sequence. Requires constant physical cues to weight shift during gait or loses balance.

Balance must be specific and described in sitting or standing, with or without support, type of support; or during a particular movement task or activity such as gait, rising from a chair, or reaching. Also describe the patient's ability to incorporate spatial relationships during movement.

EXAMPLE

Patient is able to perform bilateral activities to both the right and left of midline.

Describe behavior or painful reactions during specific movement tasks and the movements that aggravate or relieve pain.

EXAMPLE

Patient experiences sharp, severe pain in L knee with initial attempt at one-leg stand.

Pain When documenting a patient's pain, use numbers from standardized scales for rating pain, a faces scale (smile versus frown), or any of the other measurement scales such as the Oswetry. The 0/10 to 10/10 scale is most commonly used to indicate no pain to the most severe. It is important to note areas of pain, and levels at rest and during activity, as well as what relieves the pain and what increases it. The Oswetry Scale is a good indicator of how pain impacts function.

AUTHOR'S NOTE

No matter how well you qualify and describe a patient's pain, if pain does not impact function, physical therapy will not, beyond a very brief period, be medically necessary.

Describe patient's expression of sensory and temporal qualities of pain in response to tests of provocation or during rest or movement tasks.

EXAMPLE

Patient reported stabbing pain with deep friction massage that lingered for 20 minutes after completion of treatment of the R biceps tendon.

Give location of tender or trigger points and determine sensitivity with a pressure point gauge, or verbiage such as the following criteria for tenderness to touch of tender or trigger points:

0 = none

1 = mild, expressed, but no withdrawal

2 = moderate, expressed plus withdrawal

3 = severe, immediate exaggerated withdrawal

4 = patient untouchable, withdraws without palpation

Somatosensory To measure and document a patient's somatosensory functions, describe the patient's expression of sensation during sensory testing. This includes light touch, pain (sharp/dull), deep pressure, hot and cold sensitivity, and proprioception or kinesthetic sensation.

EXAMPLE

Response to light touch is absent in L side, putting patient at risk for injury.

Document the patient's ability to describe position of body part with eyes closed (proprioception), to identify objects by touch only (stereognosis), to identify use of objects (praxis), neglect of body part, and expression of sensation in absent body part or phantom pain sensation.

EXAMPLE

Proprioception of L foot is impaired, impairing safety in stand and during gait.

Unable to identify coin, comb, or pin placed in left hand.

Patient unable to determine use for cane. Patient experiences severe phantom pain in L residual limb that limits all mobility.

Cranial Nerve Integrity To evaluate and record the patient's cranial nerve integrity, describe provoked and unprovoked eye, tongue, and swallowing movements. It is also helpful to list the patient's visual field and hemianopsia and describe ability to form facial expressions and evaluate the strength of applicable cervical muscles. To complete the cranial nerve integrity evaluation, describe the patient's vestibular problems, such as nystagmus, vertigo, and past-pointing.

Posture   The patient's posture should be recorded and evaluated for the following positions: sitting, lying, standing, and during functional activity. In some cases, posture alone may be the cause of all the patient's problems and the source of their solution.

EXAMPLE

Patient demonstrates flexed posture in unsupported sitting, with inability to correct secondary to trunk weakness, perceptual deficits, etc.

In describing a patient's posture, include limb position, joint limitation, tone, and positions of comfort.

EXAMPLE

Patient's standing posture when relaxed shows forward head, knee hyperextension, and pronated feet.

The posture evaluation should also include descriptions of muscle imbalances in relation to the vertebral curves (the cervical lordotic curve, the thoracic kyphotic curve, the lumbar lordotic curve, scoliosis).

EXAMPLE

Lordotic curve is flattened, cervical lordosis increased. Include the functional implications.

Mobility   When evaluating a patient's mobility, it is important to consider all applicable aspects and types of mobility, including bed mobility, transfers, gait, wheelchair mobility (manual, electric, or powered vehicles). For babies or toddlers, the ability to creep, crawl, and cruise should be documented.

Describe assistance required by the patient in terms of the effort the patient is exerting, rather than the exertion by the physical therapist. The terms minimal assist (or limited), moderate assist (extensive), maximal assist (extensive), and total assist are commonly used. To better define these subjective terms, a percentage of effort scale serves as the basis of the FIM (Functional Independence Measures, taken from the Uniform Data System which is available from: Data Management Service, Buffalo General Hospital, SUNY at Buffalo, 100 High Street, Buffalo, New York 14203). These percentages are related to the terms as follows:

Total assist (extensive assist) = patient exerts 0% of total effort

Maximal assist (extensive assist) = patient exerts 25% of total effort

Moderate assist (extensive assist) = patient exerts 50% of total effort

Minimal assist (limited assist) = patient exerts 75% of total effort

Contact guard = patient requires hands on guarding in the event assist is needed

Supervision or Standby assist = patient has safety issues and requires someone close by for safety and occasional verbal cues

Independence = patient is able to perform activity without assistance. If a device is used it must be identified and may be considered modified independence.

The most important components of mobility are bed mobility, transfers, gait, and wheelchair mobility. Bed mobility documentation should include descriptions of rolling left or right with or without bedrails, positioning self cephally or caudally, shifting body/body segments left and right that are pertinent to a particular patient.

There are many types of transfers with multiple components. Break down the components of these functions to be specific. There are many small goals to be identified and achieved before an end result is evident. Include those components that are applicable to your patient. The following words and phrases should be used to describe transfers:

- Sit to stand, with or without pushing with arms
- Stand to sit/sit to stand
- Stand and pivot
- Partial stand to pivot with or without a device
- Full stand to pivot
- Sliding board and standing disk utilization
- Use of mechanical lift or assistive device
- Sit to supine with side-lying vs. roll then sit (long sit)

The direction of the transfer must also be described, such as transfers to the left or the right or both directions as indicated for the needs of patient.

Although there is normal variation in motor planning for transfer and mobility activities, any posturing or reflexes, weakness or other impairments that interfere with the patient's activity must be addressed in the documentation and intervention.

Gait Gait assessment and training are unique to physical therapy. They are highly skilled services, making it imperative that documentation refer to the normal phases of gait and describe deviations. Any use of a device, including assistive gait devices, prosthetics, or orthotics must also be included.

The following terms should be used to describe the gait:

Traditional	**Rancho Los Amigos**
• Arm swing	Arm swing
• Heel strike	initial contact
• Foot flat	midstance
• Toe off	terminal stance
• Swing	preswing/swing

- Width of base
- Cadence
- Stride length
- Posture
- Weight bearing/weight acceptance/weight shift
- Level of pelvis
- Stability of hips and knees
- Leg length discrepancy
- Varum or valgus in the LEs
- Assistive devices, prostheses, or orthoses required
- Distance, directionality
- Ability to sequence
- Surfaces and elevations negotiated

Whether temporarily or permanently using a wheelchair, instruction in use and determining the ability to maneuver, and type and adaptations are skilled services. The following phrases should be used to describe wheelchair mobility:

- The patient's ability to propel the chair in multiple directions for distances over varied surfaces and elevations, indoors and outdoors
- Patient's ability to manipulate the parts (i.e., brakes and armrests, etc.)
- Chair model selected (including power, scooters) and its fit
- Ability of caretaker to manage the chair, including pushing, folding, braking, and car transfers
- Ability of patient/client to manage the chair, including pushing, folding, braking, and car transfers
- Adaptations made/needed/recommended including cushions and backs
- Ability to negotiate doors and other entrances and bathrooms/toilets
- Integumentary (skin) condition and ability to change position for protection.

Wounds The patient evaluation should also include a description of any wounds, burns, scars, open areas, rashes, lesions, discoloration, or other conditions that impact function and present risk. Open areas must be measured and described. Wound measurements may be obtained with grids, pictures, picture grids, traces of the wounds, readings from a volumeter, water injection, syringe volume, or cotton-tipped applicator inserted to determine depth. Describe drainage, odor, temperature, color, bruising, scabs, skin tears, trophic changes, turgor, pigment, and skin and scar pliability.

Peripheral Vascular When evaluating peripheral vascular conditions, describe color, temperature, skin condition, and pain resulting from ischemia or claudication.

Lymphatic Record edema measurements at selected points throughout the limb. The points for measurement must be recorded as well as the circumferential measurements at the points. When possible, compare measurements to the uninvolved limb. Avoid terms such as minimal, moderate, severe, and less than or more than. At least 3 measurements should be recorded. Lymphatic evaluations should also include descriptions of peripheral pulses (Check for their presence and describe their strength), such as LE, femoral, popliteal, posterior tibial, and dorsal pedal. Describe the color, temperature, pain, and skin condition of the patient. Record the degree of pitting edema if present, using the following scale:

- 1+   barely perceptible depression (pit)
- 2+   easily identified depression (EID) skin rebounds to its original contour within 15 sec
- 3+   EID skin rebounds to its original contour within 15 to 30 sec
- 4+   EID rebound > 30 sec[24]

Describe the rationale for and use of external elastic supports or intermittent compression, as well as lymphatic drainage and massage techniques and necessity. Describe the overall size of the body, extremity, or extremity segment and how problems with size relate to function. Describe uneven fat distribution and poor weight control, as well as abnormal size. Measurements must be objective by measuring, weighing, or volumetric displacement.

Cardiopulmonary and Endurance To record cardiopulmonary status and endurance, be as objective as possible, avoiding terms such as poor, fair, and good. Instead, describe the behaviors that led you to the subjective word. Pulse oximeter readings and vital signs should be included.

EXAMPLE

Rather than patient has poor endurance, say: Patient requires 5 minute rest after 3 minutes of therapeutic exercise, able to participate for 45 total minutes.

Establish an objective baseline from which to compare improvement in function. The following should be included in descriptions of endurance:

- Autonomic responses to activity
- Breathing patterns
- Need for supplemental O2 and volume needed
- Patient complaints in quotes
- Ability to increase treatment time or repetitions or tolerance for resistive exercise
- Rate of Perceived Exertion Scales

EXAMPLE

Patient is able to accomplish only 10 feet, minimal assist with standard walker before becoming diaphoretic. Pulse increases from 80 at rest to 120 after stand pivot transfer. After 10 reps of knee extension with a 5-pound weight, patient's breathing became shallow and rate was 50 bpm. Patient requires 5 minutes of rest for breathing to return to normal after every 5 minutes of exercise. Patient tolerates only 1 hour sitting in reclined wheelchair. Requires 2 hours bedrest after every hour out of bed.

Describe cardiac status by comparing to baseline measurements at rest to measurements during activity. Examples of words and phrases include heart rate, blood pressure, respiratory rate, and breathing pattern and O_2 saturation. Any abnormalities or complaints such as chest pain, shortness of breath, and pounding in the chest should be recorded. The pre-existing need for medications and history of medical problems, such as asthma and MI should also be included in the description. Unusual fatigue and other abnormalities must be described. Patient activity should be modified as necessary by recommending paced activity, energy conservation techniques, and rest periods. Pulse oximetry, EKG readings, and similar tests should be performed during treatment.

Describe baseline pulmonary function data to compare with data during activity as necessary. Pulmonary function data includes respiratory rate; breath sounds; congestion/cough, sputum color and consistency (if present); breathing patterns; chest deformity; unusual fatigue; difficulty breathing, abnormal breathing patterns, or chest pain. The pulmonary function data should also include paced activity and energy conservation techniques and pulse oximetry measurements (see Table 9.5 for an Endurance Scale).

Body Mechanics   To evaluate body mechanics, describe posture and movement patterns during activities of daily living (ADL), leisure activities, and work-related tasks. Abnormal body mechanics may result in pain and dysfunction. Phrases and words used to describe body mechanics include abnormal body alignment, abnormal movement patterns, and inability to perform specific movement tasks. Any adaptation of a specific movement task that is required when a change in body mechanics is not feasible. This may be the case for specific impairment related to fused spine, limb contracture, or fused or limited joint movements.

Orthotics and Prosthetics   Describe orthotics and prosthetics in terms of the need for a device based on impairment in order to facilitate function. At times, a device may be used for cosmetic purposes only, but would not require rehabilitation unless instructions in skin care and application and removal are required for same. Once

**Table 9.5
ENDURANCE SCALE
(source unknown)**

Good: Tolerates normal activity, using moderate to maximal resistance. Activity and position changes with no signs of fatigue, palpitation, dyspnea, or pain. Standing tolerance is 30 minutes.

Good–: Tolerates normal activity, using moderate resistance activity, and positional changes with only occasional or minimal fatigue, no palpitations, dyspnea, or pain increase. Standing tolerance is 15 minutes.

Fair+: Tolerates high to moderate resistive activity and position change with infrequent rest periods (20 to 30 minutes work period) and minimal fatigue noted; longer time or more resistance causes fatigue, palpitations, dyspnea, or pain. Standing tolerance is 15 minutes.

Fair: Tolerates light resistive activity for short to moderate length of times (10 to 15 minutes); needs occasional rest periods; longer time or more resistance causes fatigue, dyspnea, palpitations, or pain. Standing tolerance is 10 minutes.

Fair–: Comfortable at rest; tolerates non-resistive activity for short duration (5 to 10 minutes), needs frequent rest periods; longer time, or more addition of resistance increases fatigue, dyspnea, or pain. Standing tolerance is 5 minutes.

Poor+: Comfortable at rest; tolerates non-resistive activity for short duration (2 to 4 minutes); needs very frequent rest periods of longer time or addition of resistance to exercise causes fatigue, palpitations, dyspnea, or pain. Standing tolerance is 2 to 4 minutes.

Poor: Comfortable at rest; light non-resistive activity of brief duration causes fatigue, palpitation, dyspnea, or pain. Standing tolerance 1 to 3 minutes.

Poor–: Symptoms may be present at rest; if any physical activity undertaken distress is increased. Standing tolerance less than one minute. Source Unknown

prescribed and obtained, describe how the devices are to be monitored for fit and function, and the patient must be appropriately trained to used the device. Documentation should include gait, posture, and/or body part description with and without device; alignment of the device itself relative to the body and its impact on function; ability to perform functional tasks with and without orthosis/prosthesis and need for assistive or adaptive devices; comfort; ability to apply and remove; skin integrity as a result of wearing the device; proper fit and prescription; and ability for self-care with device.

Adaptive and Assistive Devices and Equipment   Types of prostheses and orthoses include: AFO (ankle foot orthosis); KAFO (knee, ankle foot orthosis); RGO (reciprocating gait orthosis); above the knee (AK) prosthesis; below the knee (BK) prosthesis; above the elbow (AE) prosthesis; below the elbow (BE) prosthesis; myoelectric prosthesis; lumbar supports; cervical collars; slings; and bivalve casts.

When evaluating the assistive devices, describe the devices and equipment in terms of the need for a device based on impairment and their functionality in facilitating function. Once obtained, documentation must address how devices must be monitored for fit and function, and the patient must be trained to use the device. Phrases and words for this documentation include mobility, posture, ability or inability to use the device functionally, comfort, and self-care.

Types of adaptive and assistive devices and equipment include walking aids such as walkers, canes, and crutches; wheelchairs; cushions; lift chairs; transfer disks; hospital beds; reachers; elastic shoelaces; and lap trays.

Activities of Daily Living (ADL)   Due to the multitude of activities of daily living (ADL), it is necessary to describe which ADL are addressed or identified as impaired in documentation. ADL specifically relates to self-care and function in the daily environment, but excludes work-related activities. Describe ADL in objective, functional terms that can be addressed and measured for evidence of improvement. Activities of daily living include: household chores, personal hygiene, dressing, toileting, and retrieval of articles/items.

Information about ADL may be dependent on information provided by the patient during the initial interview or through observation. ADL scales, such as the Katz and Barthel's, are helpful and standardized for ADL skills

AUTHOR'S NOTE

When the patient's main complaint is pain, it may be difficult to justify treatment unless it is related to the inability to perform ADLs. the patient's subjective description of improvement and pain relief may have to be relied on for determination of progress. Whenever possible, try to duplicate the ADL in the clinic to observe actual rather than reported performance.

Functional Capacity Descriptions of results of functional capacity testing and work hardening and conditioning programs are typically completed on standardized forms for accurate, consistent recording of the performance and behavior of patients. When preparing functional activity data, avoid personal opinion. In this area—perhaps more than any other—the PT must rely on professional opinion rather than personal conclusions because patients involved in these programs are commonly patients injured on the job who are involved with the Workers' Compensation system.

Documenting Intervention/Treatment

When documenting intervention and treatment, always be specific, using CPT codeable terms (see Chapter 5) to precede all interventions, unless the interventions themselves have codes, such as ultrasound or electrical stimulation (qualifying constant attendance versus unattended). Include where the treatment was rendered and if anyone accompanied the patient/client and for how long, and specific parameters and position for reproducibility. All verbiage used in the content section that preceded this section should be applied in context.

Improvements in impairments should be stated in relation to the functional goals dependent on that improvement. For situations in which PT was administered in the OP gym, bedside, or home, clearly identify the intervention(s): modality, therapeutic activity or therapeutic exercise. Identify the specific equipment as indicated, with specific parameters (settings), time, and patient/client position. Describe the number of repetitions, dosage, distance, quality of movement/performance, deviations from norms, and degree of assistance needed. Also list the specific area of the body treated and target tissues, problems, and purpose. Include in your listing the start and end time and the duration of the session, noting if rests were needed and if so include the length of the rest.

Include vital signs in the intervention/treatment documentation as required based on history, condition treated, and precautions. It is also important to include any occurrence out of the "ordinary" or unique to that patient. Patient condition before and after treatment, including response and effect on integument should also be included.

In the record, the PT should also describe

- contraindications and precautions and barriers, if any;
- symptom relief and improved function resulting from interventions;
- specific mode of treatment and parameters for application; and
- immediate effects of intervention in terms of change in endurance, pain, sensation, reflexes, strength, and range and quality of joint movement.

Pain Management

Pain reduction as a goal must be supported in terms of how the reduction in pain is related to change in functional performance and increased ability to perform specific movement tasks. When documenting pain reduction, it is important to relate interventions to specific goals.

The continued use of physical therapy interventions without documentation of meaningful, practical, and sustained benefits related to function is not acceptable and will not be reimbursable. Use the suggested terminology examples in your continuing care documentation as well as any progress reports to support your ongoing interventions and progress toward goals. It is not the format of the entry that matters, but the content.

Summary

Regardless of the audience for the PT documentation, the content and overall progress toward goals justifies the care given and establishes medical necessity. The therapist must convey what is known to be true relative to the need for care. Historically, although PTs can verbally describe what treatment is being rendered, including the parameters and the medical necessity of treatment, the lack of ability to communicate this in writing has proven to be challenging.

Remember to include all areas of patient/client deficits that would justify the need for skilled care to ensure the patient benefits fully from the PT. For example, a patient/client with a recent amputation required gait and transfer training with and without the prosthesis, probably wheelchair training (at least early on), training on multiple surfaces in varied environments, adaptive driving, skin care training, prosthetic care training, therapeutic exercise, extensive transfer training including car transfers, ADLs, and IADLs. If the individual is working, ergonomic assessment may be indicated as well.

A listing of all of the patient's deficits should be included to all patient care, inpatient and outpatient. Additionally, emphasis should be placed on all co-morbidities because they can potentially impact the need for skilled care and prolong the need for care. However, the key to successful documentation is not in what the therapist *knows*, but what the therapist or other designated personnel *documents*. Remember, if it is not written, it was not done. Furthermore, if it is not written correctly, it might as well not have been rendered nor recorded. Only the therapist can justify the need for care and support the need through appropriate, objective, and functionally oriented documentation.

Chapter 9 Review Questions

1. What is the primary difference between the CMS 700 form and the CMS 1500 form?

2. What activities should tests and measures focus on in the initial examination?

3. Why might it be preferable to use the 700 form for an intermediary that requires it or a reasonable facsimile?

4. Explain why strength and range of motion are best described in numbers as fractions, but tone, which can also be described in fractions is preferable in verbiage?

5. Explain rehabilitation potential in the context of physical therapy.

6. Identify two components included in muscle performance and provide an example for each.

7. Explain the relationship between safety/risk reduction and strength.

8. Explain why precautions and contraindications are necessary relative to PT intervention and their relationship to medical necessity.

9. Why is pain as the primary diagnosis (in a non-pain program) not an indication for physical therapy?

10. Provide an example of objective descriptions of:
    a. Gait
    b. ROM
    c. Balance
    d. Strength
    e. WC mobility
    f. Motor control

10

Pediatric Documentation

Documentation and reimbursement for physical therapy services when working with the pediatric population present some unique challenges. This section will address the nuances of documentation in pediatric physical therapy and billing and reimbursement issues in the context of documentation, specific to pediatric physical therapy. However, the basic context guidelines are applicable to the adult population as well.

Initial Examination

Many of the major categories for examination of the pediatric patient are the same as for the adult patient. In general, physical therapists must still evaluate range of motion (ROM), muscle tone, strength, sensation, posture, and function regardless of whether the child has a musculoskeletal or neurological impairment. However, the focus and content of each of these categories is unique for the child who has a neurological impairment. In particular, young children require increased emphasis on assessment of their developmental motor skills. This section will focus primarily on conducting and documenting the content for a developmental evaluation of an infant or young child. Pediatric clients with specific diagnoses such as spina bifida warrant a more directed examination. However, the major categories described in this chapter will serve the physical therapist well for the general pediatric population.

During the initial examination, videotaping can be both beneficial to the physical therapist as well as to the child's parent or guardian. For the therapist, reviewing the videotape may allow examination of the child's movement at a pace more conducive to reflective observation. For the parent or guardian, the videotape may be a helpful reminder of the progress a child has made, which may be difficult to appreciate otherwise. Before videotaping a session, the therapist should obtain express written permission from the caregiver. From a risk management perspective, the videotape becomes a part of the medical record and must be afforded the same confidentiality as dictated by HIPAA.

History

As with any patient/client, the history should be the first assessment. The most efficient way to obtain a history is with a form developed specifically for the parent/caregiver or legal guardian to complete prior to the first session. The therapist can then use the information to obtain clarification during initial observation. If there is a medical record available, it may indicate whether there is any history of maternal drug or alcohol abuse. However, when a medical record is not available, it may not be advisable to question a parent about this history because of the degree of parental guilt that will naturally be associated with the questions. Although the question is included in the history prototype form included for reference, the information in the history is the discretion of the facility (See Table 10.1).

Observation

Before conducting the objective tests, the therapist should allow the child to play independently without assistance. This provides the therapist with the opportunity to

Table 10.1
PEDIATRIC HISTORY

Pediatric History

Child's:
Last name: **First name:**   **Middle initial:**   **DOB:**   **Age:**

Gestational age: _____ **Gender:** ___ female ___ male

SS#:   **Tel#:**   **Address:**

City: **State:**   **Zip:**

If client is minor: name of parent or responsible party:

Telephone and address if different than minor's: **Primary language:** _____

          Second language: _____

Social : Parents are: ___ married ___ separated ___ divorced ___ single

Child lives with: _____

Does the child have siblings? _____ no _____ yes If yes, number and ages _____
Was this child one of a multiple birth? _____ no _____ yes If yes, please indicate: ___ twins ___ triplets ___ quads ___ quints

Is primary caregiver responsible for the care of others in the home? ___ no ___ yes Explain:

Dwelling: Do you have to negotiate stairs into or inside your home? ___ no ___ yes

Do you have transportation available? _____ yes _____ no

Reason for PT: Please indicate if you know the child's medical diagnosis:

Did the physician indicate there were problems? ___ yes ___ no

Did the caregiver perceive there were any problems? ___ yes ___ no

Please indicate if birth mother had any of the following problems during the pregnancy:

____ pre-eclampsia   ____ excessive weight gain : _____ pounds gained

____ diabetes   ____ dehydration

____ thyroid problems   ____ premature labor

____ edema

How many pregnancies did the birth mother have? _____   **How many live births?** _____

Did the birth mother:
Smoke during the pregnancy?

Drink alcohol during the pregnancy?

Take drugs during the pregnancy that were over the counter?

Take drugs that were prescribed?

Take dietary supplements?   **Please indicate:** _____

Please indicate the type of diet the birth mother was on during the pregnancy:

Table 10.1
(Continued)

Does the child have: vision impairment _____no _____yes If yes, describe: _____

hearing impairment _____no ___yes If yes, describe: _____

Family history. Are there any other family members with similar problems? _____yes _____no

If yes, please describe:

Please check as appropriate for each category:

Birth history	Where did the birth take place? _____hospital _____home _____birthing center _____other: Please explain:

Type of delivery: _____vaginal _____C- section Did the baby present breech? _____yes _____no

Were forceps used? _____yes _____no Was vacuum extraction used? _____yes _____no

What was the baby's birth weight?_____	What was the baby's APGAR score?	How long was the baby in the hospital? Was the baby in the NICU?
What was the baby's birth length? _____	Did the baby need ventilator support?_____yes _____no	How long was the mother in the hospital?

Please indicate any diagnostic tests the baby/child has had:

Please check as applicable	No	Yes	Describe
Respiratory Problems			
Seizures			
Muscle spasms			
Head injury			
Falls			
High fevers			
Heart problems			
Shunt placement			
Failure to thrive			
Loss of consciousness			
Dehydration			
Abnormal bleeding &/or bruising			
Abnormal growth			
Loss of weight			
Diabetes			
Thyroid dysfunction			
Urinary or bowel problems			
Gastrointestinal			
HIV			

Table 10.1
(Continued)

Wheezing, coughing during or after activity			
Agitation			
Excessive sleeping			
Allergies			
Other			
Development of child: __normal __delayed			

Recent weight changes: ___weight gain ___weight loss   **Describe:**
Recent memory or cognitive changes: ___yes ___no   **If yes, please describe:**
Medications: Prescription: **Over the counter:**
General nutrition: Is the child breastfed: now ____yes _____no   **Was the child breastfed?** _____yes ____no   **How long?**____ **Is the child bottle fed?** ____yes ____no   **Combination breast/bottle:** _____yes _____no **If on formula, what type?** _____ **Diet/dietary supplements: Please indicate if child is on solid food:** _____yes _____no **Other:**
Please indicate any other information that may be important or you wish to discuss:
The above information is accurate and true to the best of my knowledge, and I give my consent for the evaluation to be performed. **Signature of responsible party if client is a minor:** _____**Date:** _____ **Printed Name:**   **Relationship to the child:**

observe how the child moves and what the child is able and unable to accomplish motorically. In addition, it allows the child time to warm to the therapist. While observing the child, general comments about motor control and movement patterns can be recorded as observed in a designated section on an evaluation form. As with adults, general observations regarding movement as well as the history, drive the decision making for performance of specific tests and measures.

Objective Data

Information gathered while observing the infant or child move independently and while taking the history from the parent or guardian will help narrow the focus of the objective assessment. For example, if the therapist notices that the child tends to scissor (cross) the legs when crawling on the floor, the therapist will want to assess hip adductor tone for possible spasticity. Recommendations for categories of objective assessment are provided in the following sections.

State of Alertness Record in the appropriate section on the form if the infant or child is awake, happy, angry, agitated, drowsy, or exhibits stranger anxiety or separation anxiety. Because the behavioral or emotional states of the infant will affect the muscle tone and motor activity the infant exhibits, it is important to note these levels of alertness.

Asymmetries To record the asymmetry of the child, document in the appropriate section if the infant or child prefers to weight bear on one side or prefers to reach with one arm more than the other, if the child shifts weight better to one side than the other, and if the child primarily transitions (changes position) only in one direction.

Postural Alignment Recording postural alignment in a child includes documenting the presence of orthopedic deformities, rib flaring, scapular winging, cortical thumb posture, frog leg posturing, opisthotonus, ankle pronation or supination in standing, genu valgus, genu varus, genu recurvatum, hip subluxation or dislocation, scoliosis, or leg length discrepancy.

Muscle Tone Assess and document muscle tone during active and passive movement. Describe the muscle tone according to location. For example, is there a difference between trunk and lower extremity tone? If so, indicate which may be low tone compared to high tone. Document if the muscle tone is different distally compared to proximally. Muscle tone should also be quantified either using a standardized scale, such as the Ashworth or modified Ashworth scale, or with more generic terms such as mild, moderate, or severe increased or decreased muscle tone.

> Modified Ashworth Scale
>
> 5/5: Normal tone: no increase or decrease
>
> 4/5: Slight tone increase, catch and release, or minimal resistance at end of range
>
> 3/5: Slight increase in tone manifested by catch, followed by minimal resistance
>
> 2/5: More marked tone through most of the range of motion but affected part(s) easily moved
>
> 1/5: Considerable increase in muscle tone, passive movement is difficult
>
> 0/5: Affected part(s) rigid in flexion or extension

AUTHOR'S NOTE

Although the Modified Ashworth includes fractions from 0/5 to 5/5, the numbers alone should be avoided since they may be confused for strength.

Range of Motion (ROM) Both passive and active ROM should be assessed and documented objectively. The ranges should be expressed as fractions (i.e., passive hip flexion 100/140). In addition, goniometric measurements of contractures should be documented. Flexibility should be assessed for the following muscles in particular: hip flexors, hip internal and external rotators, hip abductors and adductors, hamstrings, sartorius, plantarflexors, shoulder girdle musculature, and forearm pronators and supinators.

Strength Although standard muscle testing cannot be performed in infants and young children for assessments of strength, inferences regarding strength may be made based on the child's ability to move against gravity. For example, a child who has difficulty walking down stairs may have eccentric quadriceps femoris weakness. In addition, inferences regarding adequacy of muscle strength can be made based on postural alignment. For example, a child who displays rib flaring often has weakness of the oblique abdominal muscles. Pediatric patients may present difficulty "grading" muscle movements as well. For example, assessment must be made whether the child exhibits a burst of energy to accomplish a motor task but is unable to perform the task slowly and under more control.

Sensation and Perception　　Assess and document how the infant or child responds to touch, and if any self-calming techniques are used. Also observe whether the child exhibits a strong startle response that interferes with functional skills, such as sitting independently, and if child displays any evidence of tactile defensiveness. For example, determine from the child's parents if the child dislikes walking on the grass or dislikes certain textures of food. Visual tracking and hearing should also be screened.

Skin　　Assess and document if the child has any scars, pressure sores, unusual temperature of the skin and extremities, circulation problems with the fingers and toes, or discoloration on the skin or mottling. Also check the child for the presence of birth marks or any bite marks, burn marks, or bruising that may be evidence of child abuse or neglect.

Cardiopulmonary Status　　Determine and document if the infant or child has any unrepaired heart defects and any precautions or contraindications. Indicate if the child requires oxygen or ventilator support and note the child's endurance, including any shortness of breath observed.

Reflexes and Reactions　　Assessment and documentation of the following reflexes or reactions are of particular importance with regard to functional ability: asymmetric tonic neck reflex (ATNR) and equilibrium or protective reactions in sitting and standing. The presence of any tremors or clonus should also be noted. Clonus is considered significant if it lasts for more than four beats. The muscle group exhibiting clonus should be documented.

Gross Motor Development　　Infants and toddlers should be assessed for the presence of motor milestones in supine, prone, sitting, and standing. In addition, the infant's ability to roll, commando crawl, creep on hands and knees, and transition in and out of positions should be assessed and documented. The therapist should note whether the infant or young child can perform gross motor milestones as well as the quality of the movement used when performing the milestones. In addition, each of the following should be assessed and documented as age and development appropriate: head control, quadruped, gait, stair climbing, primary method of mobility, balance in all positions, length of time able to maintain standing on one leg, running, jumping, hopping, skipping, kicking a ball, catching a ball, and use of assistive devices or orthotics.

In addition to assessing these gross motor skills, evaluating the child for patterns or trends in movement can be helpful. For example, indicate if the child exhibits difficulty initiating, sustaining, or terminating movement as an adult with Parkinson's disease might, or if the infant tends to only use the extensor muscle for moving rather than balance between the flexors and the extensors. Determine and document if there are any stereotypical movement patterns, such as scissoring gait or posturing of the arms into shoulder flexion with internal rotation, forearm supination, and wrist and finger flexion.

The physical therapist that works with occupational therapists (OT) and speech therapists (ST) also needs to screen the infant or child for difficulty with fine motor or oral motor skills in order to refer the patient for services that may be indicated but have not yet been consulted. The following sections provide suggestions for screening fine motor and oral motor development.

Fine Motor Development.　　Assess and document if the infant or child is able to reach, grasp, play at midline, cross midline, or transfer an object hand to hand.

Oral Motor Development.　　Indicate and document if the infant makes any vocalizations, if the parent or guardian is having any difficulty feeding the child (i.e., if the child gags or chokes when feeding). Determine if the young child is eating age-appropriate food, such as baby food or table food, and if there are any foods the child refuses to eat. Also determine if the child drools often or regurgitates.

Assessment

Summary Statement

After gathering the subjective and objective components of the evaluation the physical therapist must pull all of the information together to develop a summary statement of the patient's status in order to establish functionally oriented goals. One strategy for beginning the assessment portion of an evaluation is to begin with a one-sentence summary of the therapist's findings. For example, "9 month old male born at 27 weeks gestational age with history of Grade IV intraventricular hemorrhage recently diagnosed with cerebral palsy." This provides the reader a brief overview of the significance of the patient's possible impairments and functional limitations.

Problem List

Many healthcare settings also require a "problem list." In the functional outcome record, identification of the problems assists all that need access to the record by providing a clear indication of what the challenges are. In the American Physical Therapy Association's (APTA) *Guide to Physical Therapist Practice,* the Nagi Disablement Model is used to categorize the summary into pathology, impairment, functional limitations, and disabilities. Each category in the body of the evaluation documentation will contain the objective assessment. The problem need not repeat the details, but should contain the problems in a summative manner. The following is an example of a general problem list:

- Moderate increased tone in plantarflexors, hamstrings, hip adductors
- Decreased strength in abdominals
- Decreased dorsiflexion ROM
- Requires moderate assistance with posterior walker for gait training 25′

Rehabilitation Potential/Prognosis

As with adults, a statement regarding the infant or child's rehabilitation potential should be included. When rating a pediatric patient's rehabilitation potential, it is helpful to include a rationale for the rating. For example, "good rehab potential as evidenced by ability to achieve quadruped with facilitation today." The statement may also include a reference to the child's level of motivation, including an example. For example, "good rehab potential as evidenced by child's strong desire to interact with environment while observed reaching for objects and babbling to therapist."

Patients who are rated as having either "excellent" or "poor" rehabilitation potential may experience difficulty with reimbursement for physical therapy services. This results from the belief that patients with "excellent" rehabilitation potential can get better without physical therapy. In contrast, patients with "poor" rehabilitation potential are viewed as receiving very little benefit from therapy services, and therefore, declared ineligible. If the PT is setting the goals with the parents or responsible party, and has considered all relevant information, the rehabilitation potential should be successful.

Goals/Functional Outcomes

From a reimbursement perspective, perhaps the most important component of the evaluation process, is the goals section. In pediatrics, many outpatient physical therapy settings will develop specific, measurable, short-term goals and less specific or objective long-term goals. In this setting, short-term goals are designed to be achieved in one month whereas long-term goals are designed to be achieved in three to six months. Regardless of the time frame preferred in the pediatric practice setting, goals should be documented in the same fashion as physical therapy goals for adults. Goals should include what is to be achieved, the time frame for achieving it, and under what conditions or criteria. Similar to goals for adult patients with neurologic disorders, goals for pediatric patients should be listed in functional terms and should include what goals the parent or guardian has for the child. Often, this may mean listing the parent's goal as a long-term goal and using the short-term goal as components necessary to achieve the parent's goal. For example, parents of infants often state they want their child to be able to walk. This can be listed as the long-term goal and the therapist can use this as a "teachable moment" for helping the parents understand what component skills the child needs before being able to walk. At times, this may mean discussing that ambulating with an assistive device qualifies as "walking."

The following are some examples of goals for the child described in the above problem list:

EXAMPLE

Short-term goals (to be achieved in one month): The child will be able to:

1. Stand with support of walker and minimal assistance with feet flat (addresses dorsiflexion range of motion)

2. Achieve gait. Ambulate 25′ with posterior walker and minimal assistance of 25% (also describe pattern)

Long-term goals (to be achieved in 3 to 6 months): The child will be able to:

1. Play for 30 seconds in a deep squat position with moderate assistance (addresses dorsiflexion range of motion)

2. Achieve gait. Ambulate 100′ with posterior walker and contact guard assistance

---

Regardless of whether a therapist is writing goals for a child or an adult, the word "maintain" should not be used. Third-party payers will not reimburse for therapy services designed to assist a patient in "maintaining" a certain skill or ability. It is believed that "maintenance" activities do not require the skills of a physical therapist or physical therapist assistant. Instead, the therapist should write goals to indicate what the child will be able to do as a result of physical therapy and why they need to have that specific skill.

Plan/Plan of Care

When compiling all of the findings, the therapist often thinks of the techniques that can be used to help the child achieve the established goals. The "plan" portion of the evaluation should include the frequency and duration the child will be treated, any recommendations for additional consultations, such as referral to OT, speech language pathology, or an orthotist, what treatment methods will be used, and how the findings and plan will be communicated to the referring physician. Regarding treatment methods, general references indicating the focus of therapy are usually sufficient. For example, "Therapeutic exercise: instruction to parents of home exercise program and strengthening, functional activities: developmental activities, gait training," indicates what the focus of the therapy session will be. The setting for physical therapy may need to be stated as well. Indicate where the child will receive physical therapy (i.e., in the home setting, in an outpatient clinic, at day care, or at school).

Documentation of the Continuation of Care

Requirements for documentation of treatment sessions, progress notes, and progress reports vary between facilities. While some facilities require a complete note regarding the treatment session, other facilities utilize a flow sheet method of recording attendance, treatment goals for the day, and significant findings for each therapy session. Inpatient rehabilitation facilities for children may only require weekly documentation. However, from a health information perspective and medical records "rules," entries should be made for each visit. Failure to do so may result in denial of payment. As a result, it is prudent for each physical therapy practitioner to be aware of the facility's requirements as well as the requirements of the reimbursing agency.

In general, progress notes/reports may contain the following:

- date of the treatment
- functional gains or changes in status since the previous visit
- specifics regarding the treatment that was provided including any parent education or home exercise instruction that was provided
- child's response to treatment (was the child able to complete the task with assistance or was the child still unable to complete the task even with the skill of the therapist or assistant?)
- length of the session
- goals of the session
- plan for the next visit

Regardless of the frequency of documentation, physical therapists should provide regular written updates to the referring physician indicating the child's progress and the treatment plan. Similar to the initial examination, the treatment plan should include the frequency and duration of physical therapy services, the type of treatment, the treatment setting, and any recommendations for additional services or consultations. As indicated in the reimbursement section, written physician authorization may be necessary to continue therapy services.

Documentation of Summation of Care

When a child has achieved maximal outcome for a specified time, or has completed a pre-authorized number of visits, and is being discharged from physical therapy, a discharge summary or documentation of the summation of the episode of care should be completed. Ideally, a discharge summary contains a statement of all the changes and significant findings addressed in the initial evaluation. The current functional status, method of mobility, and adaptive equipment should be addressed. A statement regarding progress toward the short- and long-term goals and whether or not the goals were achieved should be included. If some goals were not achieved, reasons for modifying or not achieving the goals should be stated. The discharge summary is particularly valuable if the child requires additional services in the future as the summary serves as a record of progress gained and function that may have been lost. A copy of the discharge summary should be sent to the referring physician as well (See Appendix E for documentation guidelines).

Reimbursement

Pediatric physical therapy providers have three primary methods for obtaining reimbursement (although cash payment is also possible): Part C (Medicare) funds, Medicaid, and private insurance. A description of each of these three types of funding is provided in the following sections. Qualifications for providers, requirements for the provision of services, and procedures for reimbursement are also discussed. Table 10.2 contains a summary of the requirements for provider eligibility for each of these three funding agencies.

Part C

Originally adopted in 1991 and revised in 1997, the Individuals with Disabilities Education Act (IDEA) federally mandated requirements for the provision of early intervention services for children with disabilities between the ages of 0 to 3 years old.

Table 10.2
PROVIDER ELIGIBILITY REQUIREMENTS

Requirements	Medicare Part C	Medicaid	Insurance
Current state license	Yes	Yes	Yes
Provider application	Yes	Yes	Only for network providers
Specific provider number	State specific	Yes	Insurance company specific
Resume	Yes	Yes	Insurance company specific
Background check	State specific	Yes	No
Occupational license	State specific	State specific	Insurance company specific
Liability insurance	Yes	Yes	Yes
Specific pediatric training	State specific training modules	No	No
Contract	Yes	Yes	Yes, for network providers
Federal Identification Number	Yes	Yes	Yes or social security number for individual provider

Part C, previously referred to as Part H, allows each state to develop its own guidelines for eligibility criteria and procedures for providing early intervention services. Each state designates a lead agency for coordination and funding of early intervention services. Many states utilize the following criteria to determine if a child qualifies for early intervention services:

1. The child exhibits delay in one or more of the following developmental areas: cognitive, gross motor, fine motor, communication, social and emotional, or self-help.

2. The child has a diagnosis such as Down syndrome or spina bifida that will result in developmental delay.

3. The child is at risk for developmental delay due to state-specified factors, such as prematurity, or a congenital cardiac condition.

The specific amount of developmental delay required for eligibility is established by each state. This program is not income based. Early intervention services are available for any child who meets the eligibility requirements up until the child's third birthday. To determine eligibility of children, the lead agency for each state establishes a team of professionals to screen 0- to 3-year-old children who have been identified as possibly needing early intervention services. The team consists of the family in conjunction with some combination of the following professionals: psychologist, nurse, physician, physical therapist, occupational therapist, or speech therapist. A service coordinator from the team is designated and assigned to the family and child to assist with the provision of services as determined by the team. Ultimately, the family makes the final decision regarding recommendations that will affect their child.

The team of professionals that evaluates the child may use a standardized assessment tool for determining the presence and severity of developmental delay. There are a variety of evaluation tools that compare the child's performance with other typically developing children. The main objective for the evaluation is to determine eligibility for services under Part C.

Two of the most commonly used standardized assessment tools are the Bayley Scales of Infant Development II and the Peabody Development Motor Scales (See [25] for a comprehensive review of available standardized tools). However, specific tests or standardized assessments are not required to determine eligibility. An objective narrative therapy assessment, addressing delays is acceptable for documenting a child's developmental needs.

Following the developmental evaluation, an Individual Family Support Plan (IFSP) is written to document the treatment plan based on the results of the team assessment and family input. This plan must then be reviewed every six months in addition to an annual Individual Family Support Plan (IFSP) meeting to determine what services are still needed.

As for the setting for therapy services, IDEA mandates that services must be provided in the natural environment for the child. A "natural" environment for a child may be the child's home, day care, or other community settings.

Qualifications for Providers In order to provide therapy services for children and families covered by Part C, professionals must have the following:

1. Current state license
2. Occupational license
3. State Medicaid provider number
4. Resume
5. Liability insurance

In addition, some states require completion of training modules covering such topics as:

1. The family-centered philosophy
2. An introduction to service coordination
3. Transitioning the child from Early Intervention to public school
4. Family support planning

Professionals must agree to sign a contract to provide services to Part C clients. This contract may include a procedural safeguards statement and a memorandum describing services and methods for reimbursement. However, having appropriate credentials does not guarantee approval as a provider.

Requirements for Providing Services Once the professional has met all of the qualifications to provide therapy services, the therapist must obtain a referral from the Developmental Evaluation Intervention Team, a current IFSP, and a physician's referral for physical therapy services. Therapy services may then be provided in the natural environment consistent with that particular state's provisions. When the IFSP is updated, a recommendation for continuation of therapy services must be provided. Any changes in the services must be cleared through the service coordinator.

Procedures for Reimbursement In order to receive reimbursement for therapy services through Part C, the therapist must first bill the family's private insurance agency (if they have insurance). Similarly, if the family has Medicaid, the therapist must first bill Medicaid for therapy services. Part C is considered the last payer of all third-party payers. Following receipt of payment from the family's insurer, the therapist can then bill Part C for the remaining balance up to the allowable state Medicaid rates or agreed upon allowable rate as determined by each state. Progress notes and recommendations must be submitted when billing Part C. Table 10.3 contains a summary of requirements for reimbursement for each of the three major types of funding sources.

Medicaid

Medicaid is jointly funded with federal and state monies, with the states reserving the right to certain service reimbursement. This program is considered a state-funded health insurance plan designed for children from 0 to 21 years of age who meet certain income and disability criteria. Medicaid is administered by each individual state. Each state appoints a lead agency to manage Medicaid funding and contracts for a fiscal agent to handle provider reimbursement.

Table 10.3
REIMBURSEMENT REQUIREMENTS

Requirements	Medicare Part C	Medicaid	Insurance
Physician referral	Required or from EIP	Required	Depends on state practice act and/or insurance company
Medically necessary	Yes	Yes	Yes, for continued service
Assessment	Provided by team	Yes	Often required
Treatment plan	Yes	Yes	Often required
Progress notes	Yes	To be on file	Often required
Renewal of prescription	Annually	Every 6 months	Dictated by insurance company &/or state practice act
Re-assessment	Annually	Every 6 months	Depends on insurance company &/or as condition changes, i.e., surgery
Billing forms	CMS 1500	CMS 1500	CMS 1500

Qualifications for Providers for Medicare   The qualifications for providers of Medicaid are specific to each state. In general, in order to provide therapy services for children and families covered by Medicaid, professionals must:

1. Apply for provider status;

2. Be fingerprinted for a criminal background check;

3. Provide a federal identification number (FIN) for businesses;

4. Provide social security number (SSN) if individual provider;

5. Maintain a current state professional license;

6. Obtain an occupational license (where applicable);

7. Purchase liability insurance;

8. Obtain a business license (where applicable);

9. Have the billing agent sign the provider agreement; and

10. Obtain a group Medicaid number with individuals listed separately.

AUTHOR'S NOTE

In order to provide services to adults under Medicare, a PT or facility must also obtain a Medicare provider number.

Requirements for Providing Services   After meeting all of the qualifications to provide therapy services, the therapist must obtain a physician's referral before evaluating a child. After completing the initial examination, the therapist must submit a copy of the evaluation and treatment plan to the referring physician for signature and authorization for treatment. Treatment may not begin until the physician's authorization is received.

Each state establishes guidelines regarding the frequency and duration of therapy services. In some states, visits are approved for six months and then the patient must be reassessed with the treatment plan and frequency of therapy again submitted to the physician for authorization prior to the continuation of therapy services.

Each treatment plan must include the following information:

AUTHOR'S NOTE

The information required is the same as that included in any PT treatment plan.

- Child's name
- Child's date of birth
- Child's diagnosis
- Diagnosis code
- Name of referring physician
- Date of evaluation
- Requested period for treatment
- Assessment
- Recommendations including frequency and duration
- Short- and long-term goals
- Physician's signature and authorization number
- Provider's signature and provider number

Procedures for Reimbursement Many states provide software programs for electronic billing and electronic transfer of funds. Health insurance claim forms developed by Healthcare Finance Administration (HCFA), now the Center for Medicare and Medicaid, referred to as CMS 1500 (See Appendix C) forms, are required (as for most adult PT reimbursement). These claim forms speed optical scanning for quicker turnaround in processing and reimbursement. As outlined by each state, the current procedural terminology (CPT) codes must be used for billing. The number obtained from the referring physician's authorization of the treatment plan is needed for billing purposes. Accuracy in completion of the form improves efficiency in reimbursement. If the form is not completed accurately, it could result in a technical denial, requiring resubmission.

As with all physical therapy services, only services deemed medically necessary by each individual state will be reimbursable. Depending on the state, covered services often include physical therapy, occupational therapy, speech and language therapy, and early intervention.

For children covered by private insurance, the private insurance agency must be billed before submitting for reimbursement through Medicaid. Medicaid can then be billed for deductibles, the remaining balance (up to the Medicaid rate), or for claims that were denied.

In many states, public schools are allowed to bill Medicaid for therapy services provided at the school. All requirements for providing services and reimbursement apply. Medical necessity in an educational environment must be determined by the school district.

Insurance

Private insurance companies are governed by a state insurance commissioner. Each health insurance company outlines which therapy services are covered as stated in the individual subscriber's policies. Specific regulations contained in a subscriber's policy may include:

- Pre-existing conditions
- Waiting periods
- Deductibles
- Allowable charges
- Percent of allowable charge covered
- Co-pay
- Documentation required from the service provider

Some insurance companies require therapy providers to have company-specific provider numbers. Other companies require that therapy providers apply to become part of their "network" of providers. This is especially true in managed care organizations such as HMOs, point of service (POS) plans, and preferred provider organizations (PPOs). Therapy services that are part of a network must agree to accept a set fee or capitation as the maximum allowable charge for services rendered. This type of insurance appeals to subscribers since there are either low or no deductibles and reduced co-pay. However, if the subscriber wishes to utilize an out-of-network provider, there is often an increased deductible, increased co-pay, co-insurance, or special permission required.

Requirements for Providing Services   To provide services for private insurance companies, therapists must have a current professional license for that state. To apply to be a network provider, the therapist must have current liability insurance, an occupational license, and must submit a resume. A provider with one type of insurance with an insurer does not necessarily entitle the PT to bill for services for that company. Insurance companies may have additional requirements.

Procedures for Reimbursement   Most private insurance companies require a referral from a physician in order to provide therapy services. Some companies require an updated physician referral on a monthly basis; others require the referral be updated annually. A copy of the therapy examination may be required in addition to results of a standardized developmental assessment, written narrative addressing prognosis, short-term goals, long-term goals, and the frequency and duration of therapy sessions. Interim progress notes and recommendations may also be required. Following major surgeries or changes in the child's condition, an updated physician referral and evaluation may be required.

For many insurance companies, CMS 1500 (12/90 Rev) forms are the standard requirement. These forms must include the following information:

- Signature of subscriber on file
- Name of child and date of birth
- Child's diagnosis
- Place of service
- Subscriber's policy and/or group number
- Business tax identification number or provider number
- Address of provider
- Signature of provider or assigned designee and date of services
- Appropriate CPT codes for services rendered

Schools may also bill private insurance for reimbursement of therapy services but must have the permission of the child's family to do so. If the family refuses, the school must still provide therapy services deemed medically necessary in an educational environment.

Summary

The length of time the medical record for a child should be kept does differ from that of the adult. As litigation may be involved with a disabled child, the PT must know the regulations regarding maintaining records over time (See Chapter 7).

Although there are some differences between pediatric and adult documentation, the same basic components are required. There must be medical necessity with the need for skilled physical therapy evident in the documentation. Emphasis must be on functionally oriented goals, with justification as to why the child needs the skill if the child never developed it, or why the child needs to "reachieve" the skill if it was lost secondary to a new problem. Involvement and instruction to the caregivers must also be included. If equipment or adaptive devices are required for the child, it is the responsibility of the PT to determine if payment is available. If it is, the PT must then justify through appropriate documentation why the device is necessary.

With the exception of "play" observation the process content of the document is very much the same.

Chapter 10 Review Questions

1. Compare and contrast pediatric and adult documentation.

2. What information should a treatment plan for a child include?

3. What is Part C? How does a child qualify for Part C funding? Explain the role of documentation.

4. In pediatrics, what is the relationship between observation, assessment, and documentation?

5. Give five examples of behaviors/activities that should be assessed and documented in pediatrics, as age and developmentally appropriate.

6. Explain the concept of rehabilitation potential. Why is it better to use good rather than excellent? Why is it recommended not to use poor?

7. What are the basic elements of a progress report?

8. Describe the most efficient way to obtain a history on a pediatric patient/client. What is the purpose of the history and how does it relate to the decision-making process for the initial examination session?

9. What aged children are eligible for Medicaid funding? What is the funding source for Medicaid?

10. What is the role of the problem list in the initial examination? How much detail needs to be documented in it?

11

The Electronic Medical Record or Computerized Patient Record

Although the medical field is the most documentation-intensive industry in the world, it is the least automated. It is estimated that only 3 to 5% of those practicing in medically related professions utilize computer technology to document and manage their practice.[26] The implementation of a computer-based patient record (CPR) system is now one of the highest priorities for healthcare organizations.[27]

There are many benefits to having an electronic medical record (EMR). The most critical reason is the availability and improved access to clinical information. By having one point of entry of patient information in an organization, clinicians have access to all patient information as necessary, including demographics and the most accurate insurance information. Having accurate patient information immediately available improves communication with the patient concerning their care, and allows for better case management, team communication, and decision making. By improving the quality and readability of documentation, there is also better potential for improved reimbursement. Electronic medical records also have the ability to help streamline business processes by reducing redundant activities, and eliminating paper and forms. As paper or hard copy medical records take up large amounts of space and have the potential of being misfiled or lost, the storage of discharged electronic medical records is simpler, cheaper, easier to retrieve, and can be backed up or saved in duplicate on networks or disks.

Healthcare is a $1.1 trillion industry as of the beginning of the 21st century. It is estimated that 20% of all medical procedures are under coded, leading to reduced payment. Because documentation is integrally related to reimbursement, processes and methodologies that can maximize the potential for reimbursement should be embraced.

Conversion to EMRs may streamline documentation once users are familiar with the system. However, it does not eliminate any content required or described for manual entry and all risk principles apply.

Point of Entry

Developments in technology have provided multiple options for data entry. Most facilities have two points of data entry: the business office and clinical areas for documentation, with differing types of data depending on the source. The business office staff traditionally enters patient demographic information and initial case information on a desktop computer. There are several documentation options for clinicians, all of which are dependent on the type of system in use.

Workstation

One option for documentation is the workstation or kiosk. A workstation is usually a desktop computer that may have a printer attached. Based on the number of users, the kiosk is set up in a central location where clinicians can document information as time allows. Workstations are typically less expensive than individual PCs, have more memory, and are much more durable. Recently, new software with touch screen capabilities has become available, which can minimize typing thereby speeding up the "entry" or documentation process. This type of system can eliminate the need for transcription services and expenses, but does not streamline the documentation process or eliminate redundant activities. Because the computer is in a central location, clinicians will have to document their clinical findings and treatment on paper, and then enter the information into the computer or wait for access to the kiosk. This is not an efficient use of clinician's time and may limit productivity. Additionally, if a paper record is created before electronic entry, it actually increases documentation time. Some facilities have installed individual workstations at pre-determined "desk" areas. Although this may provide each therapist a station, it may be remote to the treatment area, which decreases the efficiency because the therapist must be at the station to do the documentation.

Hand-Held Personal Data Application

Another option for documentation is the hand-held personal data application (PDA). Most PDA hardware, however, has a limited memory. Memory is discussed in terms of read only memory (ROM), or the amount of memory used for storage of documents and programs and random access memory (RAM), the amount of memory available to open and run programs. Current PDA systems have approximately 32 megabits of memory with 64 megabits of RAM, and will only support a "thin" client application, which will be discussed in the next section. The limited amount of memory can limit the clinician's ability to generate Microsoft Word or Excel documents and access the Internet and e-mail. PDAs do allow clinicians the freedom to carry the PDA with them and document anywhere, thus helping eliminate possible redundant data collection and entry. Most PDAs have touch screen capabilities, but do not necessarily have a keyboard if data needs to be typed in, although keyboards can be added to some. This can prevent the input of pertinent information, or significantly limit the quality of documentation.

The most effective and efficient alternative for electronic documentation is the laptop computer (Figure 11.1). Laptop technology has improved in recent years, with enhanced screen image quality, ability to run at faster speeds and allow for more memory, and are smaller and more lightweight. The latest laptops can weigh between two and six pounds, making it fairly easy for a clinician to carry them and document while they are seeing patients. Most computer companies offer hard drive capabilities (ROM) in excess of 40 gigabits, which enables a facility to document any type of client information, using programs such as Microsoft Word and Excel and access to the Internet and e-mail. Unlike a PDA, a laptop has a keyboard, which allows clinicians to document any specific information they need to include or add to formatted software templates. Some laptops have touch screen and electronic signature capture capabilities that can improve the speed of documentation and overall productivity.

System Architecture

There are several different types of applications, and platforms on which computer or electronic systems operate. One of the most common types of platforms is a SQL (structured query language) or Oracle database. These platforms utilize tables for the construction of their application, which makes extracting research data possible. Many of the template-driven systems are not built on an SQL platform, which makes extracting research type data impossible. Whatever platform an application is built on, it must be HL7 compliant in how it sends the medical records. HL7 is a data encryption method required by Medicare for electronic transmission. Most applications

Figure 11.1
LAPTOP COMPUTER

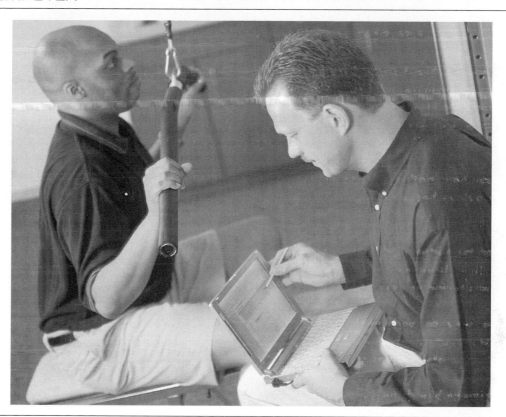

today are aware of current Medicare standards and are HL7 compliant. Generally, there are two types of environments in which applications operate. Both environments utilize a hard drive or a server for storage of medical records, but they differ in how those medical records are viewed.

Thin Client Applications

Electronic medical records reside on a hard drive or a server. Depending on the size, a large hard drive can store 80 gigabits of memory (ROM), and a large server can store in excess of 100 gigabits of memory (ROM). In a thin client environment, a medical record is never removed from the hard drive or the server. Thin client applications can be run from most types of computers, including personal data applications (PDA), because there are not large memory requirements. In this environment, a facility will view and document in a medical record while it resides on the hard drive or server. Because the patients chart is never "checked out," it is always available for multiple people to view and add documentation to. The major disadvantage to a thin client environment is if the connection to the hard drive or server is ever lost, the medical record will not be available to the clinician. All records maintained in this way should be backed up on disk.

Fat/Thick Client Applications

In a fat or thick client application, the medical record is stored on a hard drive or a server. The clinician will "check out" a copy of the medical record to complete their documentation. When the clinician has completed their documentation, they will "check in" the medical record, and update the medical record that is maintained on the hard drive or server (Figure 11.2). One benefit of this type of system is that the clinician only needs to be connected to the server or hard drive long enough to check their medical records in or out. A clinician can function off-line until they need to check in their cases. With wireless technology improvements, connecting to the server

Figure 11.2
SAMPLE OBJECTIVE DOCUMENTATION SCREEN

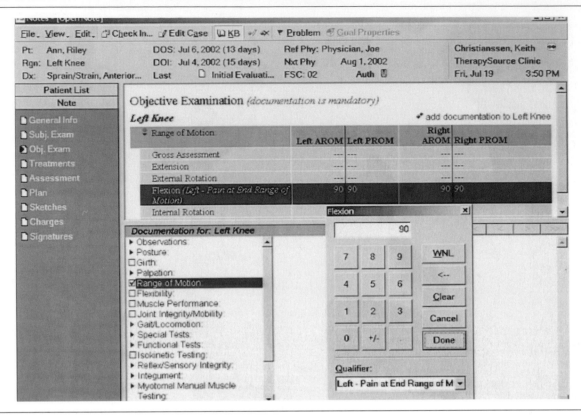

can be done via radio frequency (RF) cards rather than wired or cable systems. Network connectivity can be a concern in a fat client environment as well, but the impact will be less than a thin client environment due to the length of time a facility has to maintain a constant connection to the hard drive or server.

Training and Support

The key to successful implementation and use of hardware or software is the type of training and support a facility receives in conjunction with their equipment. The most efficient and effective software programs will quickly become ineffective if the end user does not know how to use the application. Computer and software companies usually provide some customer service and technical support for a period of time. Most companies will offer higher levels or extended coverage for an additional cost. These costs can be on a per usage, monthly, or annual basis. The skill level of the end users will dictate the level of customer service and support a facility requires. The area of customer service and support should not be neglected or negotiated out of a contract to save money. The facility using a system should ensure that in the event of staff turnover, remaining staff could train new staff or that system training is procured.

Training

Training is critical to successful software implementation and use. If a facility does not know how to use a software application or what it is capable of doing, they will not receive the full benefits of it. This can lead to eventual dissatisfaction with the application. Levels of training can vary from having to travel for training, on-site training, web-based training and tutorials, and manuals for self-paced education and training. Many companies, such as SOURCE Medical Solutions Inc., provide a combination of all of these types of training to meet the needs of a particular facility.

Traveling for training can be useful to eliminate distractions from everyday clinical functions, but can be costly for larger facilities and new employee training. On-site training is very useful because a trainer can see how a facility operates, and provide suggestions of how their system can be best implemented into the facility's work flow. On-site training can be expensive, and cost prohibitive if a facility must bring in a trainer every time a facility needs additional training or has a new employee.

Web-based technology has improved in the last few years, making training on the Internet both informative and useful. There are several options for web-based training, usually associated with an escalating price. There are self-paced tutorials, recorded web training, and live web-based training. Self-paced tutorials are similar to viewing a slide or PowerPoint presentation, guiding you through the application. Recorded web-based training is usually a recording of a live training session. This method provides the user with more useful information, with helpful hints not available in a self-paced tutorial. Live web-based training is a live session with a trainer via the web with the added ability to call in live. This method provides the end user with live training without the expense and inconvenience of traveling.

Self-paced manuals are the least expensive method of training, and can also be the least effective method of training. The manuals will always be available as a refresher or for new employees, but will not provide a facility with helpful hints of how an application can be best implemented in a facility.

Support

The technical and professional support of an application is crucial to the overall success of the software. If the software application is not working correctly, it will have a significant impact on the efficiency and effectiveness of the staff and facility. Levels of support can vary from continuous live support to limited hours of support, to e-mail communication. Within these types of support, the level of expertise can vary significantly. Some companies will provide support strictly for mechanical difficulties associated with their software. Others will support the software and the hardware that their system runs on, while others will have clinicians on staff that can assist a facility with more legal, ethical, and clinical decision making.

Documentation

There are many different ways and types of documenting both on paper and in an electronic medical record (EMR). On paper, blank sheets may be used to document the various components of the record. There are fill-in-the-blank forms for specific types of evaluations and treatments, and there are assorted flow sheets and checklists. EMR systems have very similar characteristics and formats. There are template-driven systems that allow a clinician to fill in the blanks, and there are knowledge-base–driven systems that allow a clinician to document in any way they want. However, as with paper or manual entry, there should be consistency within a facility and therapist to therapist.

Template-Driven Systems

Custom templates developed for applications should be based on input from the facility in order to provide content and formats that are facility friendly. Although this can be costly, it may be beneficial and cost effective in the long run. Some companies make the documentation templates 'appear' customized for an individual facility, incorporating some changes into standard formats. Once the original templates are created, an EMR company will charge extra for any modification or changes to the templates. Any change request can also take a considerable amount of time to create and implement. Template-driven systems appear to be easy systems to utilize, but there are some limitations. A template is excellent if everything a clinician wants to document is available. If a patient has an unusual complaint or objective finding, a template may not allow the clinician to document that information. Because of the way information is collected, compiled, and organized in a template system, it can prevent that information from being utilized for any type of outcomes research or trend analysis. Some templates have the ability to edit in content, but it may be a custom modification with a large fee.

Knowledge-Base-Driven Systems

Knowledge-base systems are similar to documenting on a blank sheet of paper. The application has a knowledge base from which clinicians can choose what they want to include or document. Knowledge-base systems give clinicians the freedom to document any information they wish to, and they can be configured to make specific documentation mandatory. Knowledge-based applications can also be configured to complete different notes with different information, which gives the appearance of being customized. Being able to make specific documentation mandatory can assist a facility in being compliant with Medicare and other accreditation guidelines. It also facilitates conducting research on specific criteria available in the system. By having an extensive knowledge base available, clinicians can document efficiently and effectively without having to type each entry individually. Implementing and documenting in a knowledge-based application usually takes more time initially due to the learning curve, but typically has better user acceptance in the long term.

Case Management

One of the keys to managing a successful practice is the ability to manage the available resources. The primary resource that needs to be managed is the active patients. Payers manage their resources by limiting the amount of treatment visits someone may receive, the dollar amount reimbursed per visit, by capitation, or by limiting the duration of time a patient/client can be treated. If a patient is treated outside of the parameters established by the payer, the payer may refuse to pay for the treatment delivered. Therefore, it is important to have the ability to monitor the status of each patient in order to enable the clinician to make appropriate decisions concerning care. By having an easy way to monitor the active patients, a facility can manage patient care efficiently, maximize a clinician's productivity, and improve reimbursement by not treating beyond pre-authorized visits and including standard, relevant content and goals (Figure 11.3).

Productivity

Productivity is a key success factor in any business, including physical therapy. Clinicians are required to see a specific number of patients/clients per day and complete all necessary documentation within the framework of their working day. When evaluating EMR systems, the application should fit into the workflow of the practice, and assist in improving productivity. Any system that adds work or disrupts the workflow of the end users will not be accepted, and will eventually have a negative impact on productivity levels. The EMR system should be intuitive to the users, support them in documenting appropriate information, and assist with case management. If a system can provide these things, it will improve the clinician's efficiency and productivity, allowing them to spend more quality time with their patients.

Unauthorized Treatment

An anonymous saying states "You do not put gross profits in the bank, you put net revenue in the bank." Therefore, it is critical that every intervention and service that is reimbursable actually be reimbursed. By being aware of the authorization status of every patient prior to treatment, as applicable, clinicians will be less likely to perform beyond authorization time. When evaluating EMR systems, a facility should have features that assist with case management, tools to maximize reimbursement for treat-

Figure 11.3
CLINICAL REPORTS

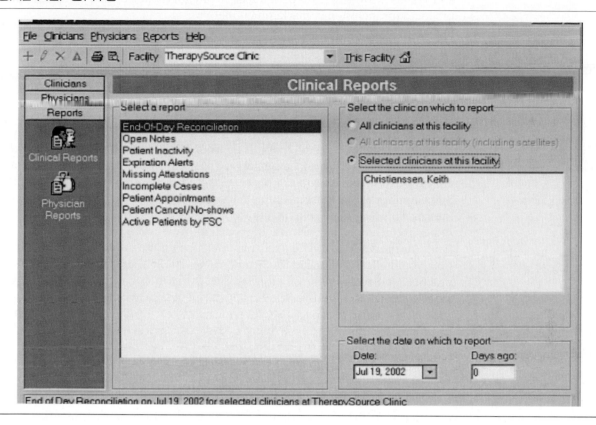

End of Day Reconciliation on Jul 19, 2002 for selected clinicians at TherapySource Clinic

ment, and alerts to inform the clinician several visits before their patient's authorization expires. By having this, the clinician can educate the patient as to their status, and take appropriate action to either discharge the patient or seek additional authorization. Knowing the status of patients allows the therapist to make better clinical decisions and provide extended care for the patients who need it.

Lost Patients

Keeping track of every active case in a facility can be difficult. If a patient/client goes on vacation for a week, or cancels appointments as a result of illness, he or she can become a lost or missing patient. Lost or missing patients mean lost revenue. An effective EMR system should be able to track patients that have not been seen in a facility for an established period of time. If a clinician is able to monitor their active cases and is alerted when a patient/client has not been seen in a set time, the clinician will be able to take appropriate action in a timely fashion. By responding to these alerts, a clinician may be able to recapture lost visits, improve facility revenues, and better assist their patients in returning to a previous level of function.

Marketing

Marketing is an important piece in building any business. Marketing helps inform referral sources of facility abilities, skills, and programs. As changes or improvements are made at a facility, it is critical to convey that information to your payers and referral sources. It is also important to monitor the referral patterns from payers and physicians, to ensure that marketing strategies are effective. Outcome effectiveness and results with a specific patient/client category can be used to benchmark quality practices for inclusion in marketing initiatives.

Physician Communication

One of the biggest challenges of any practice is keeping the referring physicians informed about their patients. The physician is accountable for all the treatment provided to their patients. It is their responsibility to oversee all the treatment given to their patients and to ensure that it is appropriate and timely. In choosing an EMR, the application must create documentation that can be produced in a timely manner, is easy to review, and provides a physician with the information they need (and want). Some applications generate template forms that may give a referral source the kind of information they need to make appropriate decisions concerning their patient's care. Other applications may provide too much information or be too "busy," making it difficult for the referral source to extract the appropriate information. The ideal application would allow a clinician to document everything that is important to their clinical practice, and to have documentation that could be provided to the referral source with only the information they want and need. Providing the physician with the appropriate information to make him or her effective and productive may have a positive impact on the amount of referrals that physician sends.

Physician Information

One part of being able to communicate to your referral sources in a timely manner is having all the physician information readily available. If a facility has one point of entry for all patient and physician information, you will be able to utilize that data for other purposes. When choosing an EMR, it is important that referral information is collected and entered into the system. By having this information in the application, you will have immediate access to the correct spelling of their name, their area of expertise, address, and phone numbers. This can make communication with a referral source quick and efficient.

Referral Patterns

One of the benefits of having an EMR is being able to look at all the data that has been entered, and use it to improve the functionality of the business. In choosing an EMR, the facility will want to have the ability to look at the referral patterns to the facility by physician, payers, and possibly by programs. If a facility has a specific program they are marketing, they will want to be able to evaluate how many referrals are being generated for that program, and how much revenue that program is producing. If a facility is spending a considerable amount of time, energy, and resources to improve the referrals from a physician or physician group, they will want to be able to evaluate their return on investment.

Another benefit of an EMR is the ability to monitor the referral patterns of the payers. Some third-party payer reimbursement rates are better than others. If a facility knows which physicians are referring patients with better reimbursable insurance, that facility could improve their net profits without having an effect on productivity by focusing their marketing on those physicians. If a facility knows which insurance companies do not reimburse well for treatment, marketing of those physicians that refer those patients could be reduced.

Business Office

One of the biggest challenges in running a business is making sure everything is organized, information is available, and that there is minimization of redundant activities. When choosing an EMR, a facility will want to ensure that the system will improve the functionality of their business, and not add more work.

Data Entry

With physical therapy as paperwork intensive as it is, one of the easiest ways to reduce redundant activities is to have one point for data entry. If there is one point of entry for information, many of the activities that are traditionally performed on a daily basis can be eliminated. Activities such as writing out charge tickets, Medicare documentation, progress, and administrative documentation can be done quickly and efficiently. By having one point of data entry, information entered once can be utilized for other purposes, such as billing, case management, marketing, and research.

Reporting

One area of responsibility for most office staff is the ability to report on the quantity of patients/clients treated, revenue generated, and money collected from co-pays (and durable medical equipment if the facility is a provider). By having this information readily available, a facility is able to quickly assess whether they are making or losing money. When choosing an EMR, a facility should be able to generate these reports quickly and easily, without having to do additional data entry.

Billing and Coding

Collecting payment for services provided is often a challenge. There are an estimated 14,000 different reasons why a payer may deny or refuse to pay a claim. Marketing can assist in getting referrals and patients, but the next challenge is getting reimbursed for services provided. Medicare and other third-party payers establish policies for what treatments they will reimburse for, and how they want bills to be submitted. Payers also aim to ensure that there is documentation to support the bills submitted for payment. In choosing an EMR, a facility should ensure the application takes the billing and coding edits into account to maximize their reimbursement. There should also be a direct objective correlation between what treatments are documented and what is being submitted for payment.

Billing and Coding Edits

Choosing the correct EMR and billing system can have a significant impact on how services will be reimbursed. It is critical that the EMR take into account the current billing and coding edits that effect reimbursement rates. There are several different types of edits that can be applied to charges. The most common types of edits are called correct coding initiative (CCI), and local medical review policies (LMRP). There are also billing rules, such as cascading, that may have an impact on how a facility submits a bill for payment. CCI edits are a Medicare part B policy that evaluates claims when two or more CPT codes are submitted for payment, to see if one comprehensive code would be more appropriate (bundling). Local medical review policies are Medicare Part A and B policies, which are administrative and educational tools used to assist physicians and providers in submitting correct claims for payment.

One billing rule that can have a significant effect on a reimbursement for services provided, are cascading rules. Currently, cascading rules only apply to some workers' compensation carriers. Under these rules, the payer will reimburse 100% of the first code submitted, 75% of the second code, 50% of the third code, and so on down the line. Therefore, how a facility submits their claims will have a significant impact on their reimbursement.

Electronic Billing

Billing software is utilized to enable a facility to electronically submit claims to a payer for reimbursement. Since many payers are moving toward electronic claims submission, it will become critical that facilities have the ability to submit their claims electronically. To minimize redundant data entry and eliminate data entry errors by the office staff, an EMR should have a billing system associated with it, or be able to interface with a billing system. By having an EMR that communicates with a billing system, the compliance with CCI and LMRP edits will be consistent, and will allow evaluation of the billing rules that need to be applied. This communication with a billing system will also ensure consistency between what has been documented and what is being billed.

Outcomes and Research

Medicare and many workers' compensation providers are requiring that clinicians have functional documentation to support continued care. The *Guide to Physical Therapy Practice* discusses proper documentation and recommended examination, tests and measures, and interventions. As the PT profession moves forward, there will be a greater demand for functional outcome-oriented documentation and research to justify what we are doing (evidence-based practice). When a facility evaluates EMR systems, the system should be evaluated on the ability to document functional problems and goals in addition to traditional impairment-based findings, consistent with the disablement model. The system should have the ability to generate PT diagnosis, medical diagnosis, and treatment-related research data, while preserving patient confidentiality consistent with all laws.

Functional Treatment

Although the trend among payers is towards functional problems and goals, it is critical that providers be able to communicate to the referral source in language that makes sense to them. When evaluating an EMR system for documentation abilities, a facility should look at its ability to generate previous and current levels of function, systems data, and traditional and functional goals with appropriate intervention and prognosis. The EMR should also have all types of treatment and functionally oriented activities to enable the clinician to make an accurate assessment of a patient's progress. The EMR should also have functional documentation for discharge planning, so that a clinician can document and demonstrate improvements and recommendations for additional levels of care as indicated.

Diagnosis-Specific Research

The practice of physical therapy has been considered as much an art as it is a science. Emphasis is being placed on evidence-based practice, rather than doing something because it has worked in the past. The need for evidence-based practice has placed a need for more research. When a facility is evaluating EMR systems, it evaluates it for its ability to generate outcomes based on medical and PT diagnosis. With the ability to generate outcomes research, a facility can establish and justify treatment protocols specific to that facility or organization. This type of research could also be utilized to contribute to the evidenced-based practice initiative being driven by the American Physical Therapy Association. Outcomes research is also an extremely useful tool when marketing a practice to payers or referral sources.

Treatment Duration Research

The ability to perform research based on treatment duration significantly impacts the origins of facility's business. It can also be a good predictor of future business. If a facility is able to generate average or below average treatment durations by diagnosis, payers and referral sources might direct more patients to that facility. Efficiency and outcomes are rewarded with more business. If an EMR system can generate reports showing the average visits for a particular diagnosis or payer, a facility could determine future staffing needs and potential revenue numbers. Choosing the correct EMR system can assist with research, marketing, and the budgeting process.

Legal Issues

There are many legal aspects in the day-to-day operations of a physical therapy business. When evaluating an EMR system for a facility, one should make sure that the application follows Medicare guidelines for documentation, takes into consideration CCI and LMRP rules, and is compliant with HIPAA regulations. There are also federal and state guidelines that need to be monitored. Finally, there are insurance credentialing procedures that need to be followed to maximize reimbursement. Many EMR systems can assist a facility with monitoring licensing and credentialing, and can ensure that a clinician's documentation supports all of the current billing rules. By implementing an EMR system that keeps current with the legal aspects of documentation, a facility can improve overall productivity and maximize reimbursement.

License and Documentation Compliance

Every clinician must have graduated from an accredited school, passed a national board examination, and maintain current licensure. Each state also has guidelines of who can legally document in a medical record. It is critical that a facility monitor each employee's credentials, when they expire, and who is documenting in the medical record. If a clinician does not maintain appropriate credentials, the clinician and facility could be liable for any problems that arise from a patient or payer. An ideal EMR systems would also have the ability to assist you in record maintenance and restrict privileges based on credentials (Figure 11.4).

Risk Mitigation

In the past, making certain errors was a mistake, but now making certain errors is considered fraud. Examples include overbilling and billing for treatment that was not actually rendered. It is a continual challenge to keep track of all the Medicare policies, CCI and LMRP edits, and Health Insurance Portability and Accountability Act (HIPAA) patient privacy requirements. All facilities must be compliant with HIPAA regulations and policies. One way to reduce your exposure to fraudulent activities is to implement an EMR that is compliant with current Medicare policy, incorporates CCI and LMRP billing rules, and is HIPAA compliant. When evaluating EMR systems, a facility must ensure that the system will reduce their exposure to fraud and risk, rather than making day-to-day activities more challenging to monitor and control.

Figure 11.4
CLINICIAN LIST

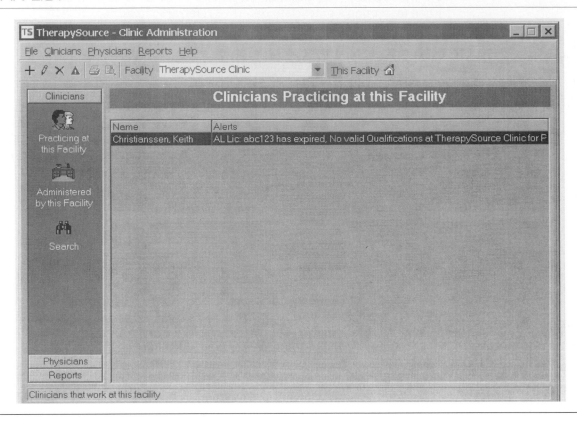

Authorized Providers

Many payers require credentials from each individual providing care to their patients. In order to maximize the reimbursement for each treatment, a facility must ensure that a credentialed therapist provides the treatment for each patient covered by a particular policy. By determining which therapists are authorized to treat a patient when scheduling, a facility will maximize each clinicians schedule and improve their productivity. Some payers, such as Civilian Health and Medical Program-Uniformed Services (CHAMPUS), do not reimburse for care rendered by physical therapy assistants (PTAs). When evaluating EMR systems, a facility should be able to control which therapist can treat a specific patient. In this way, they can maximize reimbursement for care.

Summary

There are many benefits to using electronic medical records. However, there are multiple aspects to consider before implementing any system. There are three primary considerations in evaluating any software application. First, is it going to improve the workflow and functionality of the practice? Second, is the application going to improve productivity, case management, and reimbursement? Third, is the application going to improve compliance and practice management? Once an application meets a facility's basic criteria, the next steps to evaluate are training and customer support. Training and support are the key to user acceptance and obtaining maximum benefit from the system. After a system is implemented, there will be a learning curve before complete user acceptance and improved productivity. With practice and dedication to the system, the rewards of effective and efficient documentation, increased productivity, and increased revenues can be realized.

Chapter 11 Review Questions

1. What constitutes fraud in the medical record?
2. Explain the legal issues of the EMR
3. Compare and contrast the EMR with a hard copy record.
4. Compare and contrast thick and thin applications.
5. Explain a CCI edit and how EMR can be of benefit.
6. Compare and contrast the benefits or workstations versus laptops for EMR.
7. What is the key to user acceptance and obtaining maximum system benefit? Defend your answer.
8. How can an EMR system assist in identifying potential unauthorized treatment?
9. What are the three primary considerations when considering software?
10. What is the relationship between an EMR system and evidence-based practice?

12 Utilization Review and Utilization Management

Introduction

Documentation is the means of communicating information from the professional to all "users" and "readers" of the medical record. It is the "what" therapists do and "how" it is performed. It is imperative to clearly and concisely communicate only the information that is relevant and necessary about care provided and the resulting condition of the patient or client.

As defined by the APTA, "Utilization review (UR) is a system for reviewing the medical necessity, appropriateness and reasonableness of services proposed or provided to a patient or group of patients. This review is conducted on a prospective, concurrent and or retrospective basis to reduce the incidence of unnecessary and or inappropriate provision of services. UR is a process that has two primary purposes: to improve the quality of service (patient outcomes) and to ensure the efficient expenditure of money."[28] To further break this down, the goals are:

- Delivery of cost effective high quality physical therapy services
- Identification of inappropriate or less effective and less efficient services with corrective action
- Assurance of compliance with accreditation and licensing guidelines
- Ensuring the continuum of care in a timely manner
- Assurance that medically necessary care was delivered
- Avoidance of unnecessary care beyond goals, beyond point of progress
- Delivery of service not indicated in plan
- Service not rendered for problems identified
- No baseline level of care provision based on information provided
- Referral(s) to other practitioners when out of the therapist's scope of "expertise" by training, experience, or otherwise
- Risk management (prevention of all types of loss)
- Appropriate physical therapy personnel provided care for level of skill required or by virtue of third party payer requirements.[29]

Prospective review, somewhat of an oxymoron, may also be referred to as Utilization Management (UM). UM is based on the information derived from the review process both internal and external to the organization providing services, to ensure quality of service and effective and efficient delivery.

UR is considered a component of quality assurance and may be referred to as Utilization Review Quality Assurance (URQA). In organizations or facilities with ongoing quality improvement or quality assurance programs and monitoring, URQA is often used for monitoring.

Before 1965, UR was largely experimental and not done by many providers. Medicare introduced a new era in accountability with a requirement for all hospitals participating in Medicare and Medicaid programs to also form UR committees and develop written UR plans. Initially the programs were not successful because the focus was on the fiscal portion of care, the interpretations were inconsistent, and coordination of benefits was often nonexistent. In 1972 the advent of professional standards review organizations (PRSOs) primarily for physician services occurred. PRSOs employed non-physicians and physicians to review the appropriateness and quality of medical services. Although non-physicians performed the initial review and could affirm care, only a physician could deny services. Little was done with rehabilitation review however, the focus instead being on the medical aspects. Hospitals were required to subscribe to a concurrent review and care evaluation program. This process was the precursor to the eventual development of critical pathways in the 1980s and early 1990s associated with the growth of managed care.

PRSOs evolved into peer review organizations (PROs) in the early 1980s, concurrent with the advent of Medicare inpatient Diagnostic Related Groups (DRGs), with a continued focus on medical services. Based on the Tax Equity Fiscal Reform Act, "they (PROs) monitor both quality and utilization."[30] The PROs emphasized retrospective reviews with standard pre-established review criteria based on professionally recognized treatment standards versus the concurrent review stressed by the PRSOs.

With the early growth of managed care organizations such as HMOs and PPOs, as well as hospital-based DRGs in the mid 1980s, there was an increased interest in productivity standards versus quality of care issues for physical therapy and other rehabilitation services. As a result, as organizations focused on therapist productivity versus quality of care, therapists practicing in the 1980s experienced some of the first denials for physical therapy services for Medicare beneficiaries. As costs to the Medicare program increased (due to cost shifting as a result of diagnostic related groups [DRGs]), Medicare UR was expanded to include outpatient and skilled nursing facility physical therapy services under the Part B system. This evolved from the Medicare initiative for improvement in efficiency, effectiveness, and medical necessity of care in the hospital inpatient arena. Application of UR by Medicare created added financial risk for physical therapists and organizations providing Part B services.

The practice of UR was not exclusive to Medicare. Coincident to the rise in Medicare denials for services, private payer sources looked to the Medicare system for cost containment measures. Application of UR practices facilitated examination of medical necessity, effectiveness, and efficiency of care with maximization of outcomes. As a result of therapists needing to justify care through documentation for reimbursement, evidence-based practice is being purported by the APTA. In the 21st century, as costs for healthcare continue to grow exponentially, the rise in the interest of evidence-based practice is a result of the need for justification of care. By engaging in UR and UM practices, therapists should be able to justify care by clearly identifying medical necessity and documenting efficient and effective quality care. These practices can also provide outcome data to support efficacy of intervention and the concept of evidence-based practice.

Internal UR/UM Practices

Internal UR and UM practices are based on review of documentation. The therapist must know for whom they are writing, what information must be conveyed, and the purpose for which the information will be used. From a UR perspective, the purposes include: reimbursement; effective and efficient utilization of internal resources, such as staff to monitor productivity; determination of staffing needs; consistency of content in the record; consistency and objectivity of goal setting; and effective and efficient selection of interventions and outcome data established by individual therapists. The way the information is recorded should be the same regardless of the purpose of the review. This is a principle of health information management as described by the American Health Information Management Association (AHIMA). An organization, as part of an ongoing quality management program, can review the content of the medical records for compliance. Concurrent and retrospective reviews can be utilized to ensure concurrent compliance, confirm content is legally admissible, revise guidelines for the future, develop clinical pathways, ensure effective and efficient care and outcomes, and provide educational input to staff for improvement in documentation process and content.

Utilization Review and Reimbursement

From a reimbursement perspective, the documentation must present a clear picture of the episode of care. The elements in the record that must be reviewed are: the prescription (required by Medicare, but may not be necessary with direct access or other payers); the information included for the initial examination and evaluation; all examinations performed and the objective data, documentation of continued care; and documentation of summation of episode of care (See Appendix E).[31]

Evidence of continued or continuing care includes documentation of intervention or services provided and current patient/client status, and documentation of re-examination. Colloquially, these entries are referred to as treatment notes, progress notes/reports, and periodic summaries (i.e., monthly, weekly, or as designated by policy). They can also be reflected in flow sheet format or variations of checklists and additional entry.

Documentation of summation of the episode of care occurs at the termination or discontinuation of therapy services for a specific episode. Termination or discontinuation may occur for a variety of reasons and must be clearly documented for UR purposes. Based on the APTA definitions, termination of care occurs when a patient or client has met the established PT goals. However, discontinuation may result from a variety of reasons, such as lack of progress, illness, hospitalization, patient noncompliance (with very specific descriptions of what led to this conclusion), excessive absenteeism, inappropriate patient behavior, physician decision, decision of third-party payer, or decision of a case manager. Noncompliance in this context is lack of patient compliance with instructions, thus impeding progress in an effective and efficient manner. Prolonged illness that prevents participation in scheduled therapy must result in discontinuation. However, recovery and renewed ability to participate can result in resumption of care, although if more than one or two weeks have passed and the physical status has changed, it may be considered a new episode of care or require a revised plan of care and communication with the physician (if not a self-referral).

The documentation should emphasize the disability and function versus impairment, as defined in the Nagi Disablement Model. The impairments are the pathological and physiological consequences of the disease or injury process. The functional limitations are the inability to perform a task in an efficient or competent manner as a result of the impairments. The relationship between the impairments and functional limitations should be clearly identifiable in the documentation as justification for care and appropriateness of intervention.

The review process takes each document included and examines it for relevancy to the whole picture of the patient's functional needs versus the current functional status. Because this is often based on the level or function of the patient prior to the "recent" functional change, it is imperative to clearly indicate the prior level of function in the initial examination and evaluation process. If an episode of care has ended, or the review is occurring at any point in time during the episode, the information contained in the initial report should be similar in structure and content to allow easy comparison of data. It is important to identify the reason for the referral, whether the examination concurs with the reason for referral (as indicated by the physician) and what the therapist's evaluation of the patient's potential for responding to therapeutic interventions will be. When considering the reason for referral, a clear indication should be made of the medical diagnosis versus the physical therapy diagnosis. Depending on the reason for care, they may be the same or different.

There are technical components that can be addressed with an overall review as described in detail in the APTA *Guidelines for Physical Therapy Documentation,* General Guidelines section (see Appendix E).[32]

Initial Examination and Evaluation/Consultation

The review of the examination and evaluation/consultation is performed to establish that the documentation provides clear, cohesive data that supports the evaluation conclusions. It is important to review each document/section as to its relevance to the patient/client management. This documentation should include a clear statement regarding the method of referral (self-referral in states and settings that allow for direct access or a referral from another practitioner). If the review is being performed by a third-party payer or by an internal representative, the meaning of all content must be evident.

Initial Episode of Physical Therapy Care

The history is reviewed to determine the patient/client's medical diagnoses and factors that may affect the length of care, frequency of intervention, or precautions necessary during the delivery of service, as well as evidence of informed consent. This will also allow the reviewer to determine if the appropriate risks and benefits were reviewed during the informed consent process. The care of the patient/client will be affected by the co-morbidities documented and the demographic information obtained in the history. The information documented in the history, such as living environment, co-morbidities, medications, caregiver, services (either concurrent or prior), and patient knowledge and expectations, will need to be interpreted in the evaluation to determine the exact effect and relationship to the overall care and specifically to the treatment plan and goals established. The specific relationship of this information to the plan of care should be clearly documented and the reviewer not make assumptions based on their experience or knowledge. The following sections illustrate the elements that should be clearly identified for sound documentation and review purposes.

Diagnosis/Date of Onset   The date of onset and medical and PT diagnoses are important both clinically and for reimbursement purposes. The diagnosis selected from the referral should reflect the medical condition that relates directly to the reason for the functional deficit. The diagnosis is the starting point for ensuring appropriate testing and ultimately, appropriate interventions and goals. It is therefore important for the reviewer to see clear documentation of the differentiation between the primary diagnosis and the secondary diagnoses. The selection of the diagnosis is based on the factors surrounding the onset of symptoms/functional problem. The onset could cross provider settings and therefore must reflect the circumstances surrounding the reason for physical therapy, as well as if the patient/client had previous physical therapy for the same condition. The reviewer may determine the diagnosis selected reflects a chronic condition or the onset of symptoms that may not reflect an acute condition. This would be a red flag to the reimbursement procedure and would require substantiation within the documentation to support the current provision of skilled service.

AUTHOR'S NOTE

If the condition is chronic, but there is exacerbation and remission, exacerbation, a change in function, or need for new instruction or intervention must be clearly indicated.

The utilization review process is key for ensuring that the supportive documentation is in place because this drives the documentation process for reimbursement purposes and internal decisions regarding appropriateness of services. The documentation must reflect why specific skilled intervention at this time is critical to the patient/client's functional status.

Secondary Diagnoses/Comorbidities The review includes consideration of the secondary diagnoses/comorbidities as these can affect the selection of and response to therapy. The documentation should reflect the complexity of the medical conditions pertinent to the therapeutic process. The complexity of the medical condition is often omitted and can prevent the review process from accurately assessing the true needs of the patient/client.

EXAMPLE

Referring diagnosis: Medical: Fx R hip/ORIF, NWB R × 6 weeks
PT Diagnosis: orthopedic gait abnormality, functional decline, weakness
Medical history: CAD s/p CABG × 3 years, HTN

Medications

Documentation of the patient/client medication regime is important to the review process because it can affect the interventions performed during the patient/client care. Utilization review should ensure that the medications and their complicating effects to the therapeutic process are clearly documented. Once identified the reviewer should look for the precautions and modifications to the treatment interventions that are related to the medications identified.

EXAMPLE

Medications: atenolol, lasix, dalmane
Note: monitor pulse (observe for physical S&S of distress as atenolol-beta blocker, will keep pulse lower than otherwise expected), monitor for need to urinate (lasix), schedule mid to late morning (dalmane–for sleep)

Demographic Information

The relating of the demographic information such as age, gender, date of birth, primary and secondary languages, living environment, family/social support, and potential discharge plans/destinations can effect the rehabilitation potential. The reviewer should see those items that are relevant to the delivery of service and any additional services (referrals) that may be required to address the patient/client desired outcomes. A patient/client living alone in a home with stairs and the bathroom on the second floor has very different needs than a patient living in a one-bedroom apartment on the ground floor of an apartment building. These should be evident in the documentation of the history.

History of Prior Treatment

A patient's history of prior treatment may include prior intervention for the same diagnosis by physicians, chiropractors, therapists, or adjunctive treatments. This history can support the rehabilitation potential for return to prior function. It is important to relate what has benefited the patient/client in the past and/or current episode of care, especially in the prior therapy interventions for the exacerbations of the same diagnosis. However, if the interventions were primarily palliative without active patient/client involvement, although they may have helped, they may result in denial. The utilization of previously unsuccessful modalities and interventions would be hard to support. Utilizing interventions that have been successful are easily supported, as the reasonable expectation would be substantiated by the prior response to the treatment. If no treatment has been given for this diagnosis or if it is a new problem, documentation of that can be beneficial as well. If the condition is recurring or episodic in nature, the reviewer may also look for instruction in techniques that may alter the potential for recurrence or exacerbation.

Diagnostic Testing and Examination

Documentation of the performed diagnostic testing and examination assists in the determination of medical necessity and the rehabilitation potential of the patient/ clients. All appropriate categories should be included with objective findings. Reducing data to numbers, in fraction format as possible, is universally understood.

Cognition

Recording data on the cognitive ability of the patient is often a difficult task for the therapist. However, it is extremely important to the utilization review process and can, when well written, justify the necessity of the frequency and duration of the program determined by the therapist. Documentation of confusion or disorientation is often done in a vague manner and lacks sufficient information to determine the appropriate utilization of services. No reimbursement source would want to reimburse for services given to a patient/client who is unable to follow the therapeutic program. Most therapists document orientation with a person, place, time scale, or statement of ability to follow a number of step directions. This can be augmented using the type of direction; verbal, tactile, or visual with the time needed to respond to the directions given. Appropriate utilization of services may need to be expanded due to the skill required to determine and present the appropriate stimulus to elicit the desired response. Local medical review policies and many payers have established guidelines that may limit coverage for certain diagnoses that affect cognition. These guidelines may require short interventions with more frequent assessments to clearly justify the appropriate utilization of services. In these cases providing documentation that the patient/client has appropriate cognition or easily follows multi-step directions is important to assure the reviewer that the cognitive status will not interfere with the rehabilitative process. Cognitive statements may not be required for diagnoses that do not have an effect on the cognitive status of the patient/client, such as orthopedic or industrial health patients.

Patient/Client Goals

It is important to the utilization reviewer to note the patient/client goals in order to determine, as the treatment progresses, that the therapist and patient/client are working toward the same outcomes, utilizing the appropriate interventions to achieve the results desired by the patient/client, and that they are reasonable in the context of care. The therapist may need to include family and/or caregivers in the discussion of anticipated goals to ensure the compliance with interventions and home programs as family members or caregivers may need to be involved in the administration of these.

Professional Terminology

Although the language used in the medical record must indicate the need for skilled care and should be expressed in verbiage that is professional, it must also be universally understood. Choice of word combinations can influence reimbursement and determination of medical necessity. (See Tables 12.1 and 12.2 for a list of nondescriptive and descriptive phrases and common PT terms and their functional phrase alternative.)

Examination of System: What the Reviewer Needs to See

The review of the tests and measures in any examination should identify the link between the information gathered in the history to specific tests and measures determining baselines for precautions and limitations. The reviewer should be able to discern the relationship between the selection/appropriateness of the tests and measures and the problems identified, including impairments and the resulting functional limitations and disabilities. The examination should include documentation of the physiological and anatomical status of the cardiovascular/pulmonary system and vital signs. Including vascular signs are not consistently seen as important across provider venues, but can be significant in monitoring the response to interventions and therefore baselines done at the time of the examination (especially when there are co-morbidities such as cardiac or respiratory conditions listed in the history that may necessitate monitoring).

The interpretation of the relevance and significance should be documented and the limitations/precautions identified for the safe performance of functional activities.

Table 12.1 NONDESCRIPTIVE AND DESCRIPTIVE PHRASES	Nondescriptive Phrases	Descriptive Phrase Alternative
	1. Poor quad contraction	Per manual muscle test right quadricep strength is poor.
	2. Patient unable to balance unsupported in sitting	Patient exhibits sitting balance loss to the left and posteriorly when reaching for objects and requires contact guard assistance to correct.
	3. Ambulation: Distance is improved from 30 feet to 200 feet × 3 in hallway	Neuromuscular electrical stimulation applied to facilitate strengthening exercises. Patient uses one crutch for safe gait due to knee buckling. Gait training with rolling walker and supervision of 1 for 200 feet × 3 (previously 30 feet with minimal/moderate assistance for balance). Base of support and stride length within normal limits without verbal cueing (previously moderate verbal cueing required).
	4. Patient currently complains of a constant ache in the low back radiating into the right lateral leg, right anterior thigh, and right shin	Patient reports a 10, on a scale of 1 to 10, regarding pain in the low back radiating through the right lower extremity. Patient states difficulty falling asleep secondary to low back pain.
	5. Initially, PROM R extremities WFL's, LLE: hip ext −20°, knee extension −20°; presently, ROM R extremities WFL's, LLE: −20° hip extension(s), −20° knee extension(s)	Static stretch performed within patient tolerance to improve hip extension for rolling. Pain monitored. Passive range of motion right lower extremity is within functional limits. Left hip and knee extension −20° (previously −30°).

SOURCE: Baeten, Moran, and Philippi (1999).

Table 12.2
COMMON PT TERMS
AND FUNCTIONAL
PHRASE
ALTERNATIVES

Common PT Terms	Functional Phrase Alternative
Ambulated/Walked	Gait training
Confused	Attention span deficit
Debility/Deconditioning	Functional strength deficit
Declined	Functionally regressed
Did not appear to understand	Following ____ minutes of training demonstrated inconsistent . . .
Difficulty walking	Gait deviation
Endurance	Functional activity tolerance
Helped	Facilitated
Improved	List comparative data such as: Presently ____ (Previously ____)
Observed/monitored	Evaluated/Analyzed
Pacing of activity	Instructed in energy conservation techniques
Patient unable to	Patient exhibits . . . . (describe)
Performed lower extremity exercises	Performs individualized lower extremity exercise program emphasizing
Poor gait	Gait abnormality or gait disturbance
Practiced	Instructed
Reminders	Verbal cues
Some drainage	Indicate specific amount
Stable	Beginning to respond
Stays in bed	Bed confined
Strengthening	Progressive resistive exercise
Walked	Ambulated or gait trained
Water-pik™	High pressure irrigation
Weakness	Strength deficit
Went to doctor	Transported to physician's office

SOURCE: Baeten, Moran, and Philippi (1999).

This requires the skills of the therapist to determine the specific and individualized program that will safely progress the patient/client to their desired outcomes. The tests and measures expected in this area include aerobic capacity measured objectively during functional activities or standardized exercise protocols, cardiovascular and/or pulmonary signs and symptoms and the response to increased oxygen uptake in exercise or functional activity, ventilation/respiration, and physiological responses to positional changes (i.e., orthostatic hypotension). Borg's perceived exertion scale is a good example of an acceptable measure.

Integumentary

The presence of skin integrity issues can often lead to significant compensation of function. The utilization may be impacted based on the severity, size, and location of the change in skin integrity. Many skin integrity issues also indicate a loss of sensation locally or regionally. The loss of sensation can significantly impact the patient/client's ability to perform functional activities in a safe and effective manner, necessitating teaching compensatory strategies.

Musculoskeletal

Range of Motion and Muscle Performance

These categories of examination indicate the patient/client status of range of motion, flexibility, strength, joint integrity, presence or absence of atrophy and symmetry of the body (height and weight and other anthropometric measurements may be included as well). Strength can be measured manually by manual muscle testing or instruments developed for the same purpose. Regardless of the numbering system the therapist uses, clear documentation must be made of the strength in numbers versus verbiage.

EXAMPLE

Kendall System: expressed in terms of the fractions for baselines and goals of strength

Normal	5/5
Good	4/5
Fair	3/5
Poor	2/5
Trace	1/5
None	0/5

EXAMPLE

Range of Motion Scale from the American Academy of Orthopedic Surgeons:

Shoulder Flexion Active 180°

Knee Flexion 135°

Cervical Rotation 80°

Neuromuscular

The reviewer will be expecting the measurement of tone, motor control, and the way in which the patient/client accomplishes gross coordinated movement such as balance, gait, transfers, transitions, and the coordination of these activities. The tests and measures expected to be seen in this area include use of assistive and adaptive devices, CNS integrity, cranial and peripheral nerve integrity, motor function including dexterity, coordination, agility, neuromotor development and sensory integration, pain, posture as related to position and gravity, and reflex integrity. The relationship to self-care and home management, work, community, and leisure integration or reintegration should appear in the problem summary.

The tests and measures should be carefully chosen to clearly and objectively establish the decline in function seen by the therapist and should be apparent to the reviewer to support the frequency and duration selected. The measurements should be documented in consistent terminology throughout the examination and should reflect standardized testing methods. Utilization is supported by the comparison of the results to the age-appropriate norms (See Modified Ashworth Scale, Chapter 9).

Documentation of the Continuation of Care

Colloquially called progress notes, treatment notes, or progress notes/reports, continuation of care documents are reviewed to determine the continued need for skilled intervention. The documentation provides the comparative data to justify the skilled physical therapy services rendered and should reflect measurable, functional progress (progress notes/reports). The documents may have different formats, however, all need the same identification information and basic content, regardless of format. The documentation should contain all available information to relate the skill required.

Each visit or encounter should be documented and authenticated with the applicable signature and professional designation. This is typically the therapist signature with license held followed by the license number (e.g., Patricia Smith, PT # 12345).

Documentation of supervision for treatment provided by physical therapist assistants is essential to denote the services were provided under the direction of a physical therapist. Omitting the license number may lead the reviewer to question whether a licensed therapist or assistant provided the treatment. While it seems a small issue this can lead to a technical denial of payment when the third-party payer requires treatment be provided by or under the direction of a licensed physical therapist.

Patient/client self-report should be included only as relevant to the care of the patient/client or the response to interventions. The utilization could be affected by statements documented either positive or negative reports. If the statements documented are negative, prognosticating statements such as "I don't see anything happening" or "I'm not making progress" service will likely not be viewed as appropriate. The positive, prognosticating statements such as "I am able to bathe myself now" or "I can get my hand over my head now" would support continued services based on the plan established. The reviewer will look for indications that the patient is an integral part of the review of goals and progress and would expect to see this reflected in the subjective statements documented.

Identification of specific interventions in objective, codeable terms is also important. The documentation in this section is one that can create the greatest challenge for the therapist. There are two areas affected during the utilization review of this section. The first is the correlation of the modalities and procedures given to the billing submitted to the third-party payer. These documents must match. The modalities also must adhere to the guidelines of the third-party payer in terms of covered services and should be accompanied by the appropriate physician's order for them to be recognized as billable services. Changes in treatment strategies will be reviewed for compliance to the required physician approvals necessary to comply with the procedures for each payer source. The reviewer also looks to see if the treatment strategies are relevant and effective for the problems identified and if the strategies are causing the expected progress as outlined in the goals. A lack of progress, should it be evident, would prompt the reviewer to look for alternative treatment strategies or goal revision to be implemented in a timely manner. The expectation of the UR is that the modalities rendered correspond to the services billed, that they are within the coverage guidelines established by the third-party payer, and that they are effective for the problems identified in the plan of care.

Changes in patient/client status as they relate to the plan of care, adverse reactions to the interventions, and factors that affect the frequency or intensity of the interventions and progression toward goals are usually documented as part of the assessment section. Content should reflect the thought process of the therapist and should relate the objective information documented with the patient/clients response and how that impacts the progression toward the stated goals. The assessment of the interventions given and the effect they have on the patients progress relative to function, are the only justification allowing UR to support continued treatment. This provides support for third-party payers to continue to reimburse for the services rendered. Documentation can support changes in modalities/procedures, frequency/intensity, and continuance/discontinuance.

Communication and consultation with other healthcare providers and family/ significant other/patient is also reviewed for the development of patient-oriented goals and the coordination of interventions to meet those goals. It is important to see that all healthcare professionals are working in concert to achieve the goals established and that there is no duplication of services between the providers.

Documentation of Reexamination

Reexamination, also called recertifications by some providers and Medicare, is necessary to support continued interventions beyond the original period certified (allowed) by the third-party payer. This documentation may also require physician approval to be accepted by some third-party payers.

To effectively advocate for the patient/client, the reexamination by the physical therapist should assess the effectiveness of the plan given, state the changes to be implemented and the expected outcomes based on the changes made. The documentation should also reflect the positive prognosticating factors supporting the revised plan of care including all interventions and outcomes to be carried over from the initial examination/evaluation. Revisions to the plan may be necessary to change modalities or procedures based on patient/client progress, adverse response to modalities originally planned or new medical problems occurring during the delivery of service. Patient/clients with multiple co-morbid presentation may require modifications to their plan as their co-morbidities may alter the response to treatment and, although every effort should be made to account for this at the time of the evaluation, there may be extenuating circumstances that effect the response. It is through the reexamination that physical therapists can advocate for the unique needs of the patient/client to achieve the desired outcomes that may fall outside the established parameters of the third-party payer standard guidelines.

Documentation of Summation of Episode of Care

Termination of care falls into two general categories: (1) the patient/client met the goals and expected outcomes or (2) the care was discontinued as a result of a change in the patient/client desire, medical condition, financial resources, or ability to benefit from intervention as based on the therapist's determination. Regardless of the reason for discontinuation of care the documentation should include a summary of the care from start to finish. Among the items that should be listed are the length of episode, number of visits, the current physical/functional status, the degree of goals achieved or not achieved, complications during the provision of service, and the discharge/discontinuance plan, including any written or verbal directions related to the patient/client's continued care such as home programs, referrals, follow-up physical therapy, family/caregiver training, and equipment provided.

This report should provide the justification for the skilled intervention from the last progress report. It must also justify the overall progress made from the beginning of care and why this progress could only be made through the interventions provided. The therapist should also indicate the expectations for the carryover into the home, work, or play environment and the potential for retaining the achieved functional improvements. The reviewer's ability to determine reasonableness of the plan of care is dependent on the therapist clearly and briefly documenting what happened during the course of treatment.

Utilization Management

Utilization management is the establishment of policies that minimize the occurrence of denial of payment. This starts from the moment a patient/client walks into the facility. It is important to have policies that will establish important demographic and identifying information with what information is to be verified and who will perform that part of the information gathering.

Proactive UM should include need for and presence of a correct prescription (unless self-referral in direct access states). The policy should address all applicable guidelines, including state and federal, for your setting, with compliance to the strictest regulation. As of fall 2002, Medicare requires a physician prescription to bill for services. Billing for Medicare patients requires a prescription from a physician licensed in your state.

The referral process is important as it is from this point the patient/client enters your practice. The prescription should have an order for physical therapy evaluation, a medical diagnosis that relates to the reason for the problem, and any specific information the practitioner needs to relate to you regarding the patient/client treatment. The prescription may specify a body part and the treatment of any other part without physician approval would precipitate a denial. It is therefore necessary for the therapist to carefully review the prescription and assess the problems to ascertain if further discussion with the physician is necessary. States with direct access allow the provision of therapy services without a prescription. However, billing third-party payers may require a physician referral to receive payment for PT services.

Ensuring payment also requires the determination of the primary payer and verifying that insurance is active and the extent of the coverage the patient/client is entitled to. Patient/clients often are lost in the legal language of the insurance policy and may need direction to determine the extent of coverage. This can become a tangled process and result in significant delay if not outright denial, if done after the treatment has begun. With the changing networks and insurances, it is necessary to know what contracts are current and which types of policies are accepted at a facility. Insurance companies have multiple products and each may require its own contract to become a provider. A therapist could have a valid contract with a company's Preferred Provider program and not with the HMO program. It is important to look at or copy the patient/client's insurance card both front and back. Calling to verify insurance or having direct data access can benefit both the patient/client and the provider and most insurance cards have customer service and verification phone numbers on the back of the card. The verification process can allow you to determine if there are co-payments or out of pocket expenses that need to be met and if there are limits on the number of visits per year. A facility that is not a provider may be able to receive payment but would need to assist the patient/client in verifying the insurance allows for out-of-network benefits. Although the cost may be higher than in-network, the patient/client may elect to utilize this option. Some insurance companies require pre-authorizations. This means the PT must request permission to evaluate and treat the patient.

The determination of the primary insurance is dependent on the reason for referral. One of the common mistakes made by a therapist is to verify the health insurance only to complete the history taking in the examination and determine the major complaint is due to an auto accident. If the patient was in an accident, there may be other insurance that should be billed first (i.e., personal injury protection, automobile insurance [PIP] or homeowners). Payment from these would take precedence over the individuals' health insurance until the policy is exhausted or it is determined no litigation is pending. Knowing the correct insurance to bill can avoid delayed payment or no payment at all. With insurance verified, provider number in hand, and examination/evaluation completed, you are ready to submit the billing. However, pre-authorization does not guarantee reimbursement.

External Review

This phase of the review process is performed after the claim is submitted for reimbursement to the insurance company. It is done for two purposes: to assist in the improvement of quality and service delivery, and to ensure the efficient expenditure of monies. To make this determination, external review organizations employ a variety of non-licensed and licensed staff. It is important to know who reviews your documentation as the claim is processed and what degree or experience they have.

AUTHOR'S NOTE

If all efforts are made to ensure appropriate documentation content, justification for skilled services and elimination of technical errors, regardless of who the reviewer is, the record should withstand any review.

Utilization Review Organizations (UROs) typically use nurses for the review/screening process. If the claim is questionable, a physician would review for approval or denial. There is, however, an increasing number of UROs employing nurses for denial-level decisions or employ high school graduates without medical experience to review services. The federal Government Accounting Office (GAO) reported that 67% of UROs allow nurses to shorten the length of stay for patients, 62% allow nurses to convert inpatient to outpatient services, and 28% allow nurses to shift care to another provider. The experience of the nurses is varied and can range from new graduates to nurses with years of experience in the rehabilitation setting. Knowledge of who reviews the documentation you submit may help you determine the expectations. While a relationship with the reviewer is positive, many facilities deal with multiple UROs and can only rely on general expectations. The expectations of any reviewer are to read a clear, legible document that relates the therapist's efforts to resolve the patient's problems in a timely and efficient manner. The documentation should answer, not create, questions. The focus of the review is on effective use of the dollars spent. UROs that employ nonprofessionals to perform the reviews usually give a short (3-week) training about interpretation of medical reports and claims administration. The documentation for this review needs to clearly identify what the problem with the record/care is, and will request how the therapist is planning to address the problem with care or the record, and how long it will take to resolve or remedy the problems.

Decisions are made based on the available documentation and how professionally the documentation is presented. Presentation includes the legibility, organization, and meaningfulness of the documentation submitted. Documentation sufficient for a favorable decision includes a clear statement identifying the patient's/client's problem in functional terms, a reasonable treatment plan based on medical necessity, significant functionally oriented progress with measurable changes based on professional and community standards, and evidence of clinical decision making. This is also known as reasonable and necessary care. For Medicare, there are four conditions identified for reasonable and necessary care:

1. The treatment is in accordance with accepted standard of practice, with specific and effective modalities for the patient's/client's condition.

2. The documentation denotes the complexity and sophistication of the condition of the patient such that the services of a physical therapist are required to safely perform the program. For instance, therapeutic exercise for a patient with cardiac history may require the skills of a therapist to monitor the level and intensity of the exercise program while maintaining cardiac precautions.

3. A reasonable expectation that the condition will improve significantly in a generally predictable and reasonable amount of time is based on the physician's assessment after appropriate consultation with a physical therapist. If this is not the case, it is necessary to establish a safe and effective home exercise program required in a specific disease state. This would be evident if the documentation shows the patient is meeting the goals established on the plan of care.

4. The amount, frequency, and duration is reasonable for the condition and functional deficits documented. The frequency and duration should be established as individualized as the modalities used. A reviewer may see a pattern of frequency and duration that identifies the provider for a more intensive review.[33]

Patients/clients who have policies requiring pre-authorization may require advocacy through critically documented communication with the payer to receive "reasonable and necessary" treatment. Documentation of specific skilled interventions and measurable gains are necessary in each progress report and the payer may deny any visit not justified by the specific report. Requests for continuation of care would need to include the skills required to complete the rehabilitation and the specific number of visits required to accomplish the established goals. The expectation of the intermediary/carrier is that the patient/client take responsibility for their rehabilitation and, once trained in the specific technique, continue the progression on their own.

Management of unfavorable claims requires organization and attention to detail. Most third-party payers use a denial system similar to the Medicare system. Therefore, a basic knowledge of this system is beneficial. Once a claim is submitted, an unfavorable decision may result from the technical or clinical aspect. Technical denials are typically returned to the provider also referred to as RTPs. RTPs are due to incorrect identification information, claim overlap with another provider's claim for the same or similar services, the appropriate qualifier does not accompany the submission, or the intermediary/carrier does not have a record of the provider number or participation identification.

Returned claims can be avoided by taking some simple steps. The insurance verification policy of any organization should include copying the beneficiary's insurance card and verifying eligibility before starting treatment. Medicare has eligibility information online through the Direct Data Entry (DDE) system. This system allows a provider to gather information such as exact coverage, other claims currently being billed, and the status of claims. The review of claims to be submitted should also ensure that all handwritten documents are accurate for technical information, including identification numbers and completeness. Names can be a major source of technical denials. The name on the documentation should match the name on the insurance including the suffix (Jr., Sr., or III), and avoid the use of nicknames. Knowledge of the proper billing codes and value codes can also eliminate RTP. Claims may also be denied if the services provided were non-covered items. Knowing the coverage of the policy in your particular practice setting will help a provider avoid this type of denial. Additionally, it is always the therapist's responsibility to know the laws and guidelines that govern the setting in which they operate in any state or locality. These problems are easily avoided through a process of review and establishment of proper policies.

Claims can also be denied based on the intermediary/carrier determination that the service was not reasonable and necessary. This is a judgment-based decision made from the documentation submitted with the claim. The appeal of these denials serve the facility and the profession alike as long as the documentation supports that therapy was necessary for the patients condition and the patients goals were achieved in a reasonable and predictable time. The appeal is dependent on the documentation and additional supportive statements related to the efficacy of the services provided. The decision to appeal a claim must be made based on an objective review of the services delivered. The procedure should be performed only when the documentation justifies the skilled interventions and the duration of care.

The Medicare Program is divided into Part A, or inpatient services and Part B, outpatient services. The role of the therapist in preparation of the appeal may vary depending on the type of appeal. It could range from collecting and reviewing the documentation to participation in the hearing process depending on the size, personnel, and policies of the facility. Part A claims management is usually coordinated by administrative personnel and the therapist may have very little to do with the appeal. Part B (outpatient) appeals are very paperwork intensive and time sensitive. However, if there is a policy outlining the specific responsibilities of each person, the time involved is worth the potential outcome. This process allows you to defend the decisions made during the course of care and can effect future denials. The appeal allows you to advocate for all future patient/clients with a similar condition and care. Medicare has three levels of appeal: Additional Development Required (ADR), Hearings, and Administrative Law Judge (ALJ).

A level one ADR process occurs when a submitted claim has an error in the technical data. These claims are not reviewed based on medical necessity. The denial may result from a diagnosis not matching the services billed, an incorrect billing period, onset date or date treatment commenced, information crossing lines in electronic claims, incorrect name, and so on. The claim can be corrected and resubmitted for payment. The documentation must be received in the intermediary's office no later than 45 days from the ADR date. Each record should be submitted with a copy of the ADR attached. Records sent with multiple beneficiaries or multiple ADRs attached will cause delays that may result in automatic denials for lack of meeting the time deadlines. Organization and clarity is a must at this stage in the denials process.

Level two denials occur when the technical information does not support the physical therapy intervention. Examples of this are the claim exceeded the usual and expected number of treatments (with approximately 30 days used as a reference) the medical diagnosis selected did not clearly indicate the need for physical therapy or did not support the need for the PT services rendered, or the facility has been selected for a focused review and the intermediary has chosen to review all or a percentage of claims submitted. A new provider may be on a percentage review in this category to demonstrate to the intermediary their knowledge of the regulations and ability to provide care under the guidelines.

Since January 1, 2002, the percentage of claims reviewed at this level can only change after the intermediary/carrier has performed three educational seminars with the provider. These can be provided either in person or by teleconference. If the review at this level results in a denial the provider and the beneficiary receive a notice of claim determination, which gives the dates of service that were denied and a specific reason for the denial. The therapist or provider should review the documentation and determine if there is sufficient reason to appeal the claim. The benefits are not only the recovery of payment but also include education of the patient and intermediaries reviewer, validation of the treatment chosen, and the providers increased understanding of specific intermediary policy. The decision to appeal is based on three factors: if the documentation speaks to the reason for the denial; if the provider understands the payers regulations well enough to clearly explain why the treatment given fits in the guidelines stated; and lack of clear connection of all the factors for the reviewer, such as multiple co-morbidities and key symptoms related to the diagnosis. If the facility decides to appeal the claim, a letter of support may accompany the request and can include information supporting the rationale for the interventions and duration. It may not include any new or conflicting information than what was originally submitted. A checklist for the completion of an appeal letter is helpful to target the specific reason for the request. Employing resources such as the State Insurance Commission, Department of Labor, Workers' Compensation Board, Professional organizations, physicians, family members, and the patient can provide support for an appeal. A well-educated therapist and client/patient can be the key ingredients to a successful request. Using the resources and substantiating the rationale for treatment can result in a successful claim review. If the claim is denied at this level, the provider may request a fair hearing.

Fair hearings are typically conducted by telephone. However, an in-person hearing or on-the-record hearings may be requested. The provider must notify the intermediary in writing as to the type of hearing requested and the intermediary/carrier will then provide written notice of the date and location of the hearing. The notification usually includes the name of the officer hearing the cases and the claims to be discussed/reviewed. There has been concern as to the qualifications of the fair hearing officers because there is not a clear credential requirement for this position.

On-the-record hearings are conducted based on documentation and written materials submitted to the fair hearing officer. There is no verbal communication between provider and payer in this type of hearing and this is usually the least likely option. More commonly chosen options are the telephone hearing or an in-person hearing. These require considerable organization and preparation as both review specific treatments relating them to the supportive research and intermediary regulations to justify the skills of a therapist as the only discipline able to effectively provide the treatment. The phone hearing should involve the treating therapist unless not available. If the therapist is not available, then the individual designated must be familiar with the guidelines for reasonable and necessary care and have sufficient knowledge of the claim to defend it. In-person hearings allow for the presentation of expert witnesses, research articles, history of payment for similar conditions, and any other pertinent information necessary to successfully defend the delivery of service. A list of the items and witnesses to be presented as well as the résumés of each witness should be provided to the hearing officer in advance of the hearing.

Determinations can only be based on the evidence offered at the hearing and the information from the previous appeal levels. Recourse beyond this level is conducted before an administrative judge and requires legal assistance and expert witnesses are not optional. To proceed beyond the fair hearing should be carefully considered as the cost may outweigh the benefit.

Administrative Law Judge (ALJ) hearings are the last level of appeal and are considered when the hearing is unsuccessful. Larger providers who have sufficient claims and wish to set precedence in order to avoid future similar claims being denied usually select this appeal level.

If the decision of denial is overturned at any appeal level payment of the claim is made. If the decision to deny is upheld through the last attempted appeal level payment is withheld.

In summary, the therapist and all involved in the documenting and billing of services should read and understand the regulations and guidelines for all payers before initiating care. The policies and guidelines will assist the therapist in determining the patient/client eligibility and the allowable treatment modalities for each payer. The examination/evaluation provides the objective and measurable baseline data, which establishes the need for the skills of a physical therapist to carry out the plan of care and safely restore the function of the patient/client. All documentation must use consistent measures and tests that meet standard requirements with established norms for the population being treated. The progress reports must reflect the functional changes occurring as a direct result of the interventions and the critical decision making performed to alter the program as needed to achieve the goals established. This step is critical when the progress made is not as rapid as predicted by the therapist on the evaluation. If events that were not predictable at the time of the evaluation occur, the documentation could show reason to justify continued intervention. It is essential that documentation be complete, accurate, and legible for submission of a good claim. Having this allows for the therapist to appeal decisions made by the third-party payers and advocate for the patient and profession.

Summary

A reviewer must decide retrospectively if the therapeutic intervention was medically necessary, if the skilled services were required and if so, if they were required for all sessions based on the patient's progress and goals. For a concurrent review, the questions are the aforementioned as well as if skilled services will be required beyond the point of review based on the information provided. Specific forms can be developed for this purpose (See Table 12.3).

There are significant educational opportunities and benefits to having an active internal UR/UM process. This process can range from internal chart audits performed utilizing a check sheet to audits by a designated UR department. The results of a strong UR program provide the basis for a strong UM process. Adherence to policies and procedures can result in quality-oriented programs resulting in significant patient outcomes in a cost-effective and efficient manner.

According to Stern (1997), the record or the documentation of services provided will be the primary basis for determination of reimbursement.[34] The term primary is used because the reviewer may, depending on the organization, have the opportunity to question the providers or the individuals that actually provided the care. There may be records to use as baseline for prospective decision making. If the documentation reflects the medical necessity of skilled service or intervention, and if the interventions are relevant and appropriate for the PT problems indicated, reimbursement and or appropriate continued care can be justified.

Table 12.3
THERAPY CONTENT
REVIEW WORKSHEET

Reviewer: **Date:**

This is an: _____ **Internal review**   _____ **External review**

Record reviewed is for: ___ outpatient   ___ inpatient

Review is: ___ retrospective   ___ concurrent

Treatment venue:

Acute care hospital.   ___ inpatient/acute   ___ inpatient/acute rehab
_____ out-patient

SNF: ___ inpatient   ___ ___ out-patient

Rehab Hospital: ___ inpatient   ___ out-patient

_____ CORF   ___ PT in private practice

_____ Home health   ___ Out-patient

_____ Other: _____

Referral status: _____ self-referral/direct access or _____ physician: If physician referred, status of prescription: ___ in record, written ___ in record, verbal only

General information: please indicate if the item is present by writing y for yes. If missing or incorrect, please put n for no. If not applicable, please put NA.

_____ entries are in ink (single color)

_____ informed consent indicated

_____ blank spaces are not left in entries

_____ co-signature is used for student entries/or for those pending licensure

_____ each category of entry is labeled: i.e., PT Evaluation, PT notes, Discharge Summary

_____ pages are numbered as appropriate, i.e., if multipage evaluation, pages are numbered

_____ indicates release to communicate with family members, caregivers, others

_____ treatments rendered are included in the initial plan or interim plans

_____ reason(s) for treatment are indicated

_____ all required components are included

_____ all required components are identified

_____ patient response to treatment is indicated

_____ consistent attendance is indicated or follow-up is indicated for missed appointments

_____ treatment is modified based on changes in function or response to interventions

_____ outcomes/goals are expected in a reasonable time frame

_____ based on the content, care rendered was skilled

_____ based on the content, care was reasonable and necessary

_____ all entries match: billing dates, visit dates, plan, interventions, goals

_____ signatures are original or electronic

_____ entry errors are corrected appropriately

Identification:

_____ patient/client's full name   _____ date of birth, age are included
(on all pages)

_____ other identification as relevant   _____ all entries are dated/timed

_____ signatures include license #   _____ signatures include professional designation

Table 12.3
(Continued)

Initial Examination/Evaluation with Plan of Care

Please check yes or no to indicate if the item is included or is not included

yes	no	Content item	yes	no	Content item
____	____	Medical history of presenting problem	____	____	Objective measures of systems dysfunction/functional problems
____	____	Primary medical diagnoses	____	____	Problem summary/Indication of clinical judgment
____	____	Co-morbidities/concurrent problems	____	____	Objective, measurable goals that relate to identified problems
____	____	Physical Therapy diagnosis or problem	____	____	Goals are time defined by dates and days or weeks as indicated (circle which)
____	____	Precautions/contraindications	____	____	Combination of impairment and functionally based goals that are related
____	____	Barriers			
____	____	Demographic information: Psychosocial, social, and environmental concerns	____	____	Indication of patient/client/caregiver participation in goal setting
____	____	Cognition: Ability to communicate/understand	____	____	Treatment plan: Interventions in CPT codeable verbiage that matches problems and goals
____	____	Indication of patient/client's knowledge of problem or responsible party	____	____	Patient/client/caregiver educational learning goals are included
____	____	Other services patient/client is receiving related to episode of PT care	____	____	Frequency
			____	____	Duration
			____	____	Prognosis: Rehabilitation potential
____	____	Prior level of function relative to presenting problem	____	____	Authentication: PT signature and designation
____	____	Indication of collaboration with other professionals as indicated	____	____	License number

	yes	no
Does the venue require a Physician Plan of Care (POC)?	____ yes	____ no
If yes, is all the information included from the above (except objective systems data)?	____ yes	____ no
Is the POC signed by the physician?	____ yes	____ no
Is the POC dated?	____ yes	____ no
Is the POC signed on the appropriate date, prior to intervention?	____ yes	____ no

Table 12.3
(Continued)

Continuation of Care: PT treatment notes, progress notes, progress reports

There is an entry for each encounter/visit:	____ yes	____ no
Each entry is authenticated?	____ yes	____ no
Professional designation is included for all?	____ yes	____ no
License number is indicated for all?	____ yes	____ no
Co-signature as appropriate?	____ yes ____ no ____ not applicable

PT Treatment Notes (if applicable, if not, indicate NA)

Please check yes or no to indicate if the item is included or is not included

yes	no	NA	Content item	yes	no	NA	Content item
____	____	____	Each entry is dated	____	____	____	Interventions match POC
____	____	____	Time of visit is indicated	____	____	____	Equipment issued is indicated
____	____	____	Patient/client self-report in quotes as indicated	____	____	____	Instructions given are indicated
____	____	____	Indication of body areas treated	____	____	____	Response to treatment
____	____	____	Indication of procedures/ interventions rendered in CPT codeable verbiage	____	____	____	Reflects communication with others as applicable
____	____	____	Parameters of interventions included	____	____	____	Indicates if anyone else was present during sessions

Other:

Table 12.3
(Continued)

Progress Notes/Reports
Please check yes or no to indicate if the item is included or is not included

yes	no	NA	Content item	yes	no	NA	Content item
___	___	___	Each entry is dated	___	___	___	Interventions match POC
___	___	___	Time of visit is indicated if single progress note for single day	___	___	___	Equipment issued is indicated
___	___	___	If entry is for a single or combination of visit days, dates are indicated and frequency of notes is appropriate for acuity	___	___	___	Reflects communication with others as indicated, including caregivers
				___	___	___	Instructions given are indicated
___	___	___	Indicates where treatment rendered/who accompanied	___	___	___	Reflects communication with others as indicated, i.e., physicians, other team members, including phone calls, conversations, conferences
___	___	___	Patient/client self-report in quotes as indicated				
___	___	___	Indication of body areas treated	___	___	___	Reflects adjustments in plan
___	___	___	Indication of procedures/interventions rendered in CPT codeable parameters of interventions included	___	___	___	Indicates where treatment rendered
				___	___	___	Information matches previous entry information
___	___	___	Includes progress toward goals as established in initial examination/evaluation or reexamination	___	___	___	Indicates how patient came to PT
___	___	___	Response to treatment is indicated				
___	___	___	Indicates change in status				

Other:

Table 12.3
(Continued)

Reexamination

Reexam is included as applicable to evaluate progress and modify or redirect? ____ yes ____ no ____ NA

Please check yes or no to indicate if the item is included or is not included or NA for not applicable.

yes	no	NA	Content item	yes	no	NA	Content item
___	___	___	Entry is identified as re-exam, re-cert or appropriate designation	___	___	___	Need for continued skilled intervention is included
___	___	___	Timely, every 30 days or as applicable for setting (60 days, then q 30 for CORFs)	___	___	___	Elements from progress notes/treatment notes included relative to system dysfunction, functional deficits
___	___	___	Updated functional status, progress toward initial or interim goals	___	___	___	Authentication: PT signature, professional designation
___	___	___	Goals modified to reflect changes: up or down				

Other:

	yes	no
Is a recertification signed by the physician required?	___ yes	___ no
If required, is it in the record?	___ yes	___ no
If in the record, is it signed and dated?	___ yes	___ no
Does it contain progress toward goals, interventions provided, and any goal and plan revisions as applicable?	___ yes	___ no

Table 12.3
(Continued)

Summation of Episode of Care

A summation of care/discharge summary is included?   ____ yes   ____ no

Please check yes or no to indicate if the item is included or is not included or NA for not applicable.

yes	no	NA	Content item	yes	no	NA	Content item
___	___	___	Entry is identified	___	___	___	Discharge instructions to patient/client/caregivers
___	___	___	Summary of interventions				
___	___	___	Time frame of treatment: From : to	___	___	___	Indication of patient/client/caretaker instruction
___	___	___	Reference to all problems, impairment and functional addressed in initial exam/eval	___	___	___	Instructions are signed off on and copy is in record
				___	___	___	Recommendations/plan regarding condition, communication post discharge including:
___	___	___	Goals/outcomes achieved relative to initial plan and revisions	___	___	___	Referrals for additional services
___	___	___	Indication of current functional status	___	___	___	Recommendations for follow-up PT
___	___	___	If goals not achieved, indication of reason	___	___	___	Equipment provided
___	___	___	Indication that referral source has been informed or communicated with	___	___	___	Recommendation for physician follow up
				___	___	___	Indication of where discharged to
				___	___	___	Indication of why being discharged
				___	___	___	Authentication: PT signature, professional designation

Other:

Table 12.3
(Continued)

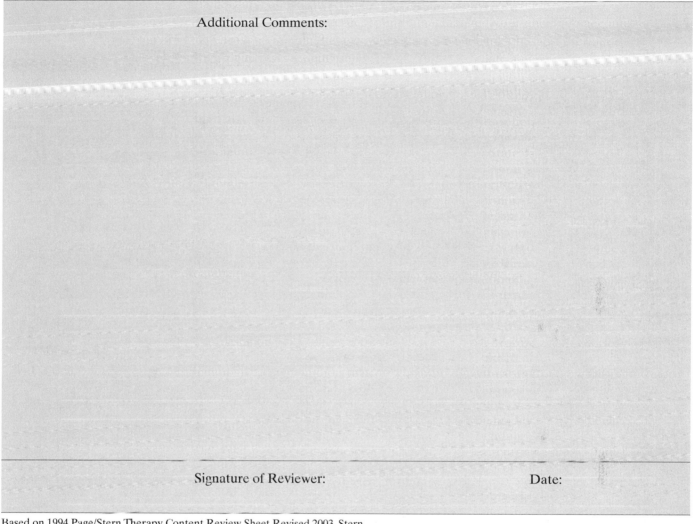

Additional Comments:

Signature of Reviewer: Date:

Based on 1994 Page/Stern Therapy Content Review Sheet Revised 2003, Stern.

Chapter 12 Review Questions

1. What is utilization review?
2. How does utilization review differ from utilization management?
3. Compare and contrast retrospective, concurrent, and prospective review processes.
4. What is the continuum of care in PT?
5. How does quality improvement or quality management relate to utilization review programs?
6. What does an external review organization base their decisions for payment on?
7. Define a technical error and give three examples. How can they be avoided?
8. Compare and contrast first- and second-level denials and their appropriate appeals.
9. Compare and contrast internal and external utilization review.
10. Explain the benefits of expressing examination findings in numeric terms.

Pediatric References

1. McEwen, I., ed. *Providing Physical Therapy Services,* Section on Pediatrics, APTA; 2000.
2. Individuals with Disabilities Education Act of 1990, 20 USC s1401.
3. Individuals with Disabilities Education Act of 1991, 20 USC s1401.
4. Individuals with Disabilities Education Act of 1997, 20 USC s1401.
5. Bayley, N. (1993). *Bayley Scales of Infant Development,* 2nd ed. San Antonio, TX: Psychological Corporation.
6. Folio, R.M., and Fewell, R. (1983). *Peabody Developmental Motor Scales and Activity Cards.* Chicago, IL. Riverside Publishing.
7. Piper, M.C., and Darrah, J. (1994). *Alberta Infant Motor Scale (AIMS).* Philadelphia, PA: WB Saunders.
8. Newborg, J., Stock, J.R., Wnek, L., Guidubaldi, J., and Svinicke, J. (1984). *Battelle Developmental Inventory.* Chicago, IL: Riverside Publishing.
9. Chandler, L.S., Andrews, M.S., and Swanson, M.W. (1980). *Movement Assessment of Infants.* Rolling Bay. WA: Infant Movement Research.
10. Russell, et al. *Gross Motor Function Measure.* Toronto, Ontario, Canada: 2002.
11. Blue Cross/Blue Shield of Florida: www.bcbsfl.com
12. Part C Florida District 3: www.elephantstoinsects.com

Appendices

Appendix A   Abbreviations

Appendix B   CMS 700 Form

Appendix C   CMS Forms 1450 and 1500 with Instructions

Appendix D   ICD-9 Code Terms

Appendix E   APTA Guidelines for Physical Therapy Documentation

Appendix F   Goal Writing Exercise

Appendix G   Note Writing Exercise

Appendix H   Documentation Content Exercise

Appendix I   Physical Therapy Note Examples

Abbreviations

Δ	change
↓	decrease
↑	increase
↔	to/from, in/out of
=	equals
<	less than
>	greater than
#	number
−	minus
+	plus
&	and
etc	etcetera
%	percentage
‖	parallel bars
@	each or at
@	at, before
°	degree
p̄	after
s̄	without
♀	female
♂	male
¶	paragraph

a	artery
ā	ante (L)
A	assistance
AA	atlantoaxial; adjusted age; active assist
AAA	abdominal aortic aneurysm
AAO X3	alert, awake, and oriented to date, person, place
AAROM	active assisted range of motion
AARP	American Association of Retired Persons
Abd	abduction
ABG	arterial blood gases
AC	alternating current; acromioclavicular
a.c.	before a meal
ACA	anterior communicating artery; anterior cerebral artery
ACCE	academic coordinator of clinical education
ACL	anterior cruciate ligament
ACM	Arnold-Chiari malformation
ACSM	American College of Sports Medicine
AD	adduction, advanced directive
ADA	American Dental Association, American Dietetics Association

ad lib	ad libitum (Latin), at pleasure
ADD	attention deficit disorder
ADHD	attention deficit hyperactivity disorder
ADL	activities of daily living
Adm	admitted
ADR	additional development required
AE(A)	above elbow amputation; preferred is transhumeral amputation
AF	atrial fibrillation, Arthritis Foundation
AFB	acid-fast bacillus
AFO	ankle foot orthosis
AFP	alpha-fetoprotein
AGA	appropriate for gestational age
AHA	American Heart Association, American Hospital Association
AHIMA	American Health Information Management Association
AI	aortic incompetence
AIDS	acquired immune deficiency syndrome
AIMS	Alberta infant motor scale
AK(A)	above knee amputation; preferred is transfemoral amputation
ALL	acute lymphocytic leukemia, anterior longitudinal ligament
ALJ	administrative law judge
ALS	amyotrophic lateral sclerosis; advanced life support
AM	morning
AMA	against medical advice; American Medical Association
amb.	ambulate, ambulation
AML	acute meylogenous leukemia, acute myelocytic leukemia
ANA	American Nursing Association
ANS	autonomic nervous system
ant.	anterior
AOTA	American Occupational Therapy Association
AP	anteroposterior, before dinner
APGAR	appearance, pulse, grimace, activity, respiration
APTA	American Physical Therapy Association
ARC	Association for Retarded Citizens
ARD	Assessment reference dates
ARDS	adult respiratory distress syndrome
	acute respiratory distress syndrome
ARF	acute renal failure; acute respiratory failure
AROM	active range of motion
AS	aortic stenosis; ankylosing spondylitis
As & Bs	apnea and bradycardia
ASA	aspirin
ASAP	as soon as possible
ASD	atrial septal defect
ASHA	American Speech and Hearing Association
ASIS	anterior superior iliac spine
Asst, assist	assistance, assist
ATC	athletic trainer, certified
ATNR	asymmetric tonic neck reflex
AV	arteriovenous; atrioventricular; aortic valve
AVM	arteriovenous malformation
B	bilateral; both
BAER	brainstem auditory evoked response (hearing screening)
BBA	Balanced Budget Act
BBB	blood brain barrier; bundle-branch block
BCBS	Blue Cross and Blue Shield

BE	barium enema
BE(A)	below elbow amputation; preferred is transradial amputation
BIB	drink
BICU	burn intensive care unit
BID	bis in die (Latin); twice a day
Bil, bilat	bilateral
BIN	twice at night
BK(A)	below knee amputation; preferred is transtibial amputation
bl	blood, bleeding
BM	bowel movement
BMI	body mass index
BMR	basal metabolic rate
BMT	bone marrow transplant
BOS	base of support
BP	blood pressure; bed pan
BPD	bronchopulmonary disease
BPH	benign prostatic hyperplasia
bpm	beats per minute; breaths per minute
BPPV	benign paroxysmal positional vertigo
BR	bathroom
BRP	bathroom privileges
BS	breath sounds; blood sugar; bowel sounds
B/S	bedside
BSA	body surface area
BT	Blalock-Taussig (shunt)
BUN	blood urea nitrogen
bw	body weight, birth weight
bx	biopsy
$\bar{c}$	with, calorie
C	centigrade cale
C & S	culture and sensitivity
Ca	calcium, about
Cal	calories
CA	cancer; chronological age
CABG	coronary artery bypass graft
CAD	coronary artery disease
CARF	Commission on Accreditation of Rehabilitation Facilities
Cath.	catheter
CBC	complete blood count
CC, C/C	chief complaint; carbon copy
cc	cubic centimeter
CCCE	clinical coordinator of clinical education
CCI	Correct Coding Initiative
CCU	cardiac care unit, coronary care unit
CDC	Center for Disease Control and Prevention
CDMM	Clinical Decision Making Model
CF	cystic fibrosis
CFS	chronic fatigue syndrome
CG	contact guard
CHAMPUS	Civilian Health and Medical Program-Uniformed Services
CHD	Congenital Heart Disease
CHF	congestive heart failure
CI	clinical instructor, curie
CICU	coronary intensive care unit; cardiac intensive care unit
CK	creatine kinase

CLD	chronic liver disease, chronic lung disease
CLL	chronic lymphocytic leukemia
cm	centimeter
CMC	carpometacarpal (joint)
CML	chronic myelogenous leukemia
CMR	computerized medical record
CMS	Center for Medicare and Medicaid (formerly Healthcare Finance Administration, HCFA), to be taken tomorrow morning
CMV	cytomegalovirus
CAN	certified nursing assistant
CN	cranial nerve, tomorrow night
CN I	olfactory
CN II	optic
CN III	oculomotor
CN IV	troclear
CN V	trigeminal
CN VI	abducens
CN VII	facial
CN VIII	vestibulocochlear
CN IX	glossopharyngeal
CN X	vagus
CN XI	accessory
CN XII	hypoglossal
c/o	complains of
CNS	central nervous system
CO	cardiac output; carbon monoxide, complains of
CO_2	carbon dioxide
Cont.	continued
COPD	chronic obstructive pulmonary disease/disorder
CORF	certified outpatient rehabilitation facility
COTA	certified occupational therapist assistant
CP	cerebral palsy, chest pain, cold pack
CPAP	continuous positive airway pressure
CPI	clinical performance instrument
CPK	creatine phosphokinase
CPM	continuous passive motion machine
CPR	cardiopulmonary resuscitation, computerized based patient record
CPT	current procedural terminology
CS	cesarean section
CSF	cerebrospinal fluid
CT	chest tube, computed axial tomography (CAT)
CV	cardiovascular
CVA	cerebrovascular accident
CVL	central venous line
CWI	crutch walking instructions
CXR	chest x-ray
D & C	dilation and curettage
DAFO	dynamic foot ankle orthosis
DC	direct current
D/C,DC,d/c	discharge, discontinue
DDD	degenerative disc disease
DDE	direct data entry
DDH	developmental dysplasia of hip
DDS	doctor of dental science

Dept.	department
DF	dorsiflexion
DHT	Dobhoff (feeding) tube
DIP	distal interphalangeal (joint)
DJD	degenerative joint disease
DLE	discoid lupus erythematosus; disseminated lupus erythematosus
DLT	double lung transplant
DM	diabetes mellitus
DMD	Duchenne muscular dystrophy, doctor of medical dentistry
DME	durable medical equipment
DNA	deoxyribonucleic acid
DNR	do not resuscitate
DO	disorder; doctor of osteopathy
DOA	dead on arrival; date of admission
DOB	date of birth
DOE	dyspnea on exertion
DPT	diphtheria-pertussis-tetanus vaccine, doctor of physical therapy
DRGs	diagnostic related groups
DT	delirium tremens
DTR	deep tendon reflexes
DVT	deep vein thrombosis
Dx	diagnosis
EBP	evidence-based practice
EBV	Epstein Barr virus
ECF	extended care facility, extracellular fluid
ECG, EKG	electrocardiogram
ECMO	extracorporeal membrane oxygenation
EEG	electroencephalogram
EENT	ears, eyes, nose, and throat
EF	ejection fraction
EFA	essential functional activities
EIA	exercise induced asthma
EID	easily identified depression
EIP	early intervention program
EKG	electrocardiogram
ELBW	extremely low birth weight
ELISA	enzyme-linked immunosorbent assay
ELS	Eaton-Lambert syndrome
EMG	electromyography
EMR	electronic medical record
EMS	emergency medical services
EMT	emergency medical technician
ENT	ears, nose, and throat
EOB	edge of bed
ER	emergency room; external rotation
ERT	estrogen replacement therapy
ES	electrical stimulation
ESR	erythrocyte sedimentation rate
ESRD	end stage renal disease
ETOH	alcohol (use/abuse)
ETT	endotracheal tube
Eval	evaluation
EX	exercise
EXT	extension, extensive

F	♀, fair, female,
f/u	follow-up
FAQ	frequently asked questions
FAS	fetal alcohol syndrome
FBG	fasting blood glucose
FBS	fasting blood sugar
FES	functional electrical stimulation
FEV_1	forced expiratory volume in 1 second
FI	fiscal intermediary
FIM	Functional Independence Measure
FIN	Federal identification number
FL	functional limitation, Florida
Flex	flexion
FOB	father of baby
FOIA	Freedom of Information Act
FOR	Functional outcome reporting
FOTO	Focus on Therapeutic Outcomes, Inc.
FSH	fascioscapulohumeral dystrophy
FSP	family service plan
Ft.	feet
FT	feeding tube; full term
FTT	failure to thrive
FUO	fever of unknown origin
Funct	functional
FVC	forced vital capacity
FWB	full weight bearing
FWW	four wheeled walker or front wheeled rolling walker
fx	fracture
G	good
G tube	gastrostomy tube
G#P#A#	number of births, pregnancies, and abortions
GA	gestational age
GAO	Governmental Accounting Agency
GB	gallbladder
GBS	Guillain-Barré syndrome
GCS	Glasgow Coma Scale
GER	gastroesophageal reflux
GI	gastrointestinal
Gm	gram
GMFM	Gross Motor Function Measure
GPCI	geographic practice cost indices
Grava	gravida = number of births
GSW	gun shot wound
gt	gait training
GU	genitourinary
GVHD	graft versus host disease
GYN	gynecology
H & P	history and physical
H	flu haemophilus influenza B, hydrogen, hour
h/o	history of
HA	headache
Hams, hs	hamstrings
Hb	hemoglobin

HBP	high blood pressure
HC	heelcords
HCFA	Health Finance Administration (now CMS)
Hct	hematocrit
HCVD	hypertensive cardiovascular disease
HDL	high density lipoprotein
HEENT	head, ears, eyes, nose, and throat
HEP	home exercise program
Hg, Hgb	hemoglobin
HH	home health, hand held
HHA	home health aide, hand held assist, home health agency
HHS	Department of Health and Human Services
HIB	haemophilus influenza B (vaccine)
HICN	health insurance claim number
HIE	hypoxic-ischemic encephalopathy
HIM	Health Information Management
HIPAA	Health Insurance Portability and Accountability Act
HIV	human immunodeficiency virus
HKAFO	hip knee ankle foot orthosis
HLA	human leukocyte antigen; homologous leukocytic antibodies
HLT	heart, lung transplant
HMD	hyaline membrane disease
HMO	health maintenance organization
HNP	herniated nucleus pulposus
HPI	history of present illness
Hs	at bedtime
HRT	hormone replacement therapy
HTN	hypertension
HO	heterotopic ossification; house officer
HOB	head of bed
HOH	hard of hearing
HP	hot pack
HPI	history of present illness
Hr.	hour
HR	heart rate
HSV	herpes simplex virus
Ht	height
HT	heart transplant
HVGS	high volt galvanic stimulation
HX	history
I	independent
I & D	incision and drainage
I & O	input and output
IADL	independent/instrumental activities of daily living
IBS	irritable bowel syndrome
ICA	internal carotid artery
ICD	international classification of diseases
ICH	intracranial hemorrhage; intracerebral hemorrhage
ICP	intracranial pressure
ICU	intensive care unit
ID	infectious disease
IDDM	insulin dependent diabetes mellitus
IDEA	Individuals with Disabilities Education Act
IEP	individualized exercise program, individualized education plan

IF	interferential electrical stimulation
IFSP	Individual Family Support Plan
Ig	immunoglobulin
IM	intramuscular
Indep	independent
inf.	inferior
instr	instructions
Imp	impression
IPA	independent practice association
IPPB	intermittent positive pressure breathing
IPO	independent practice organization
IQ	intelligence quotient
IR	internal rotation
IRB	institutional review board
ITB	intrathecal baclofen
IUD	intrauterine device
IUGR	intrauterine growth retardation
IV	intravenous
IVC	inferior vena cava
IVH	intraventricular hemorrhage
IVP	intravenous pyleogram
J tube	jejunostomy tube
JCAHO	Joint Commission on Accreditation of Healthcare Organizations
JP	Jackson-Pratt (drain)
JRA	juvenile rheumatoid arthritis
jt	joint
KAFO	knee ankle foot orthosis
Kcal	kilocalories
Kg	kilogram
KUB	kidney, ureter, bladder; kidney and upper bladder
L	left, lower
L, l	liter
l/min	liters per minute
LAP	laparoscopy; laparotomy
LAQ	long arc quad
LBP	low back pain
LBQC	large based quad cane
LBW	low birth weight
LD	learning disability
LDL	low-density lipoprotein
LE	lower extremity
LFT	liver function tests
LG	limb girdle dystrophy
LGA	large for gestational age
Lim	limited
LLC	long leg cast
LLE	left lower extremity
LLL	left lower lobe
LLQ	left lower quadrant
LMN	lower motor neuron
LMRP	local medical review policies
LOC	loss of consciousness
LOS	length of stay

LP	lumbar puncture
LPN	licensed practical nurse
LT	lung transplant, light
LTCF	long-term care facility
LTD	limited
LTG	long-term goal
LUE	left upper extremity
LUL	left upper lobe
LUQ	left upper quadrant
M	male, ♂
MAO	monoamine oxidase
max	maximum; maximal
MCA	middle cerebral artery
MCL	medial collateral ligament
MCO	managed care organization
MCP	metacarpophalangeal (joint)
MD	muscular dystrophy, medical doctor
MDA	Muscular Dystrophy Association
MDS	medical data sheet, material data safety sheets, minimum data set
MED	minimal erythemal dose
MENS	microcurrent electrical stimulation
mets	metastasis
METS	maximal
MFT	muscle function test
MH	moist heat
MHP	moist hot pack
MI	myocardial infarction
MICU	medical intensive care unit
min	minimal; minute
ml	milliliter
mm	millimeter
mm Hg	millimeters of mercury
MMPI	Minnesota Multiphasic Personality Inventory
MMR	measles, mumps, rubella (vaccine)
MMT	manual muscle test
mo	month; months old
mob.	mobilization, mobility
mod	moderate
MOM	milk of magnesia
MP	metacarpophalangeal joint (MCP), metatarsophalangeal joint (MTP)
MRE	manual resistive exercise
MRI	magnetic resonance imaging
MS	multiple sclerosis; mitral stenosis
MSDS	material safety data sheet
MT	medical technologist; metatarsal
MTBI	minimal traumatic brain injury
MTP	metatarsophalangeal joint
MV	mitral valve
MVA	motor vehicle accident
MVP	mitral valve prolapse
MWD	microwave diathermy
N	normal; nausea
N & V	nausea and vomiting
N/A	not applicable

NAD	no appreciable disease, nothing abnormal detected, no acute distress
NCQA	National Committee on Quality Assurance
NCV	nerve conduction velocity
NDT	neurodevelopmental technique or treatment
neb	nebulizer
NEC	necrotizing enterocolitis
Neg	negative (−)
NG	nasogastric
NGT	nasogastric tube
NICU	neonatal intensive care unit; neurological intensive care unit
NIDDM	non-insulin dependent diabetes mellitus
NIH	National Institute of Health
NIOSH	National Institute for Occupational Safety and Health
NKA	no known allergies
nl	normal
NMES	neuromuscular electrical stimulation
NPO	non per os (Latin); nothing by mouth
NSAID	non-steroidal anti-inflammatory drug
NSR	normal sinus rhythm
NWB	non-weight bearing
O	objective
OA	osteoarthritis
OB	obstetrics
Obj	objective
OBRA	Omnibus Budget Reconciliation Act
OBS	organic brain syndrome
OD	overdose, doctor of optometry
OHTx	orthotopic heart transplant
OI	osteogenesis imperfecta
OIG	Office of the Inspector General
OLD	obstructive lung disease
OLT	orthotopic lung transplant
OM	otitis media
OMRA	Other Medicare Required Assessment
OOB	out-of-bed
OP	outpatient
OPV	oral polio vaccine
OR	operating room
ORIF	open reduction internal fixation
OSHA	Occupational Safety and Health Administration
OT	occupational therapy, occupational therapist
OTC	over-the-counter
OTR	occupational therapist, registered
Oz	ounce
$\bar{p}$	after
P	poor, plan
PA	pulmonary artery; posterior-anterior; physician's assistant
PAC	premature atrial contraction
Para.	number of pregnancies, paraplegic
Path	pathology
PCA	patient controlled analgesic; posterior cerebral artery; posterior communicating artery
PCP	primary care physician
PD	Parkinsons disease; peritoneal dialysis

PDA	patent ductus arteriosus, personal data application
PDD	pervasive developmental delay
PE	pulmonary embolus; pulmonary edema
PEDI	Pediatric Evaluation of Disability Inventory
PEEP	positive end-expiratory pressure
PEG	percutaneous endoscopic gastrostomy
Per	by, through
PERRLA	pupils equal, round, react to light, accommodate
PET	positron emission tomography
PF	plantarflexion
Pharm D	doctor of pharmacy
PH	past history
PI	present illness
PICA	posterior inferior cerebellar artery; posterior inferior communicating artery
PICC	peripherally inserted central catheter
PICU	pediatric intensive care unit
PID	pelvic inflammatory disease
PIP	proximal interphalangeal (joint), personal injury protection
PKU	phenylketonuria
PLF	prior level of function
PLL	posterior longitudinal ligament
PM	afternoon
PM & R	physical medicine and rehabilitation
PMH	past medical history
PMS	premenstrual syndrome
PNF	proprioceptive neuromuscular facilitation
PNI	peripheral nerve injury
PNS	peripheral nervous system
PO	per os (L); by mouth
POC	plan of care
POD	post-op day number
POMR	problem oriented medical record
Pos	positive (+)
POS	point of service plan
Poss	possible
post.	posterior
post-op	post operative
PPH	primary pulmonary hypertension
PPO	preferred provider organization
PPS	prospective payment
PRE	progressive resistance exercises
Pre-op	pre-operative
Pron	pronation
PRN	as needed
PRO	peer review association
PROM	passive range of motion; premature rupture of membranes
PRSO	professional standards review organization
PSIS	posterior superior iliac spine
Psych	psychology, psychiatric
Pt., pt	patient; point, pint
PT	physical therapy; physical therapist, prothrombin time
PTA	physical therapist assistant; prior to admission; post-traumatic amnesia
PTB	patellar tendon bearing (prosthesis)
PTIP	Physical therapist in independent practice (now PTPP)
PTPP	Physical therapist in independent practice (was PTIP)

PVC	premature ventricular contraction
PVD	peripheral vascular disease
PVH	periventricular hemorrhage
PVL	periventricular leukomalacia
PWB	partial weight bearing

q	every
QA	Quality Assurance
QC	quad
qd	once daily
qh	every hour
QI	Quality improvement, quality indicator
qid	quater in die (Latin); four times a day
qiw	four times per week
qod	every other day
qt	quart
quad	quadriplegic

R	right
R/O	rule out
RA	rheumatoid arthritis; right atrium, rehabilitation agency (certified)
RAM	random access memory
RAD	reactive airway disease
RAI	resident assessment instrument
RAP	resident assessment protocol
RAS	reticular activating system
RBBB	right bundle branch block
RBC	red blood cell
RCA	right carotid artery
RD	registered dietician
RDS	respiratory distress syndrome
Re	regarding
Rehab	rehabilitation
REM	rapid eye movement
Reps	repetitions
RF	radio frequency
RGO	reciprocating gait orthosis
RLE	right lower extremity
RLL	right lower lobe
RLQ	right lower quadrant
RML	right middle lobe
RN	registered nurse
R/O, RO	rule out
ROM	range of motion, read only memory
ROP	retinopathy of prematurity
ROS	review of systems
RPE	rate of perceived exertion
RR	respiratory rate
RRR	regular rhythm and rate
RSD	reflex sympathetic dystrophy
RSV	respiratory syncytial virus
RT	respiratory therapy/therapist; recreational therapy; renal transplant
RTx	radiation therapy; renal transplant
R UE	right upper extremity
R UL	right upper lobe
R UQ	right upper quadrant

RUGs	Resource utilization groups
RV	right ventricle
RVRBS	relative value resource based systems
RVU	relative value component
RW	rolling walker
Rx	drug; treatment; therapy, prescription
$\bar{s}$	without
S	sine (Latin); subjective, supervision
S & S	signs and symptoms
S/P	status post
SA	sinoatrial
SACH	solid ankle, cushion heel
SBA	stand-by assistance
SBQC	small based quad cane
SC	sternoclavicular
SCC	sickle cell crisis
SCD	sickle cell disease
SCFE	slipped capital femoral epiphysis
SCI	spinal cord injury
SCID	severe combined immunodeficiency disorder
SCM	sternocleidomastoid
SD	seizure disorder; standard deviation
SDAT	senile dementia, Alzheimer's type
SDR	selective dorsal rhizotomy
sec	second
sed	sedimentation
SED	suberythemal dose
SGA	small for gestational age
SI	sacroiliac; sensory integration
SICU	surgical intensive care unit
SIDS	sudden infant death syndrome
SNF	skilled nursing facility
SLC	short leg cast
SLE	systemic lupus erythematosus
SLP	speech language pathology
SLR	straight leg raise
SMA	spinal muscular atrophy
SNF	skilled nursing facility
SOAP	subjective, objective, assessment, plan
SOB	short of breath
SOC	start of care date
SOMR	source oriented medical record
S/P	status post
SR	sinus rhythm
SSN	social security number
ST	speech therapy, speech therapist
Stat	immediately
Stats	statistics
STD	sexually transmitted disease
STG	short-term goal
Str	strength
STNR	symmetric tonic neck reflex
STSG	split thickness skin graft
sup	superior; supination, supervision
SV	stroke volume
SVC	superior vena cava

SVD	spontaneous vaginal delivery
SWD	shortwave diathermy
Sx	symptoms
Sz	seizure
T	trace
T & A	tonsillectomy and adenoidectomy
TA	tricuspid atresia
TAH	total abdominal hysterectomy
TAR	total ankle replacement
TB	tuberculosis
TBA	to be announced
TBI	traumatic brain injury
TBSA	total-body surface area
Tbsp	tablespoon
TCU	transitional care unit
TD	tardive dyskinesia
TEF	tracheoesophageal fistula
TENS	transcutaneous electrical nerve stimulation
TER	total elbow replacement
TES	threshold electrical stimulation
TGA	transposition of great arteries
THA	total hip arthroplasty
Ther ex	therapeutic exercise
THR	total hip replacement
TIA	transient ischemic attack
tid	three times a day
tin	three times a night
TIW	three times a week
TKA	total knee arthroplasty
TKE	terminal knee extension
TKR	total knee replacement
TLSO	thoracic lumbar spine orthosis
TMJ	temporomandibular joint
TO	telephone order
TOF	Tetralogy of Fallot
TOS	thoracic outlet syndrome
TPN	total parenteral nutrition
TPR	temperature, pulse, and respiration
Trng	training
TSA	total shoulder arthroplasty
Tsp	teaspoon
TTWB	toe-touch weight bearing
TUR	transurethral resection
Tx	treatment; traction; therapy; transplant
U	upper
UA	urinalysis
UE	upper extremity
UMN	upper motor neuron
UM	utilization management
UQ	upper quadrant
UR	utilization review
URA	utilization review organization
URI	upper respiratory infection
URQA	utilization review quality assurance

UTI	urinary tract infection
US	ultrasound
UTI	urinary tract infection
UV	ultraviolet
VA	Veterans administration, visual acuity
VAD	ventricular assistive device, vertebral axial decompression
VAS	visual analogue scale
VC	vital capacity
VD	venereal disease
vent	ventilator
VLBW	very low birth weight
VO	verbal order
Vol	volume
VPA	valproic acid
Vs	vital signs
VSD	ventricular septal defect
VT	ventricular tachycardia
W	walker
W/C, WC	wheelchair
WB	weight bearing
WBAT	weight bearing as tolerated
WBC	white blood cell, white blood count
WFL	within functional limits, within full limits
WHO	World Health Organization
WIC	women, infants, children
Wk	week
WNL	within normal limits
W/O	without
wp, wpl	whirlpool
wt	weight
$\bar{x}$	except, times
XRT	radiation therapy
Yd	yard
y.o.	years old
yr	year

B

CMS 700 Form

DEPARTMENT OF HEALTH AND HUMAN SERVICES
CENTERS FOR MEDICARE & MEDICAID SERVICES

PLAN OF TREATMENT FOR OUTPATIENT REHABILITATION
(COMPLETE FOR INITIAL CLAIMS ONLY)

1. PATIENT'S LAST NAME	FIRST NAME	M.I.	2. PROVIDER NO.	3. HICN

4. PROVIDER NAME	5. MEDICAL RECORD NO. *(Optional)*	6. ONSET DATE	7. SOC. DATE

8. TYPE ☐ PT ☐ OT ☐ SLP ☐ CR ☐ RT ☐ PS ☐ SN ☐ SW	9. PRIMARY DIAGNOSIS *(Pertinent Medical D.X.)*	10. TREATMENT DIAGNOSIS	11. VISITS FROM SOC.

12. PLAN OF TREATMENT FUNCTIONAL GOALS

GOALS *(Short Term)*

OUTCOME *(Long Term)*

PLAN

13. SIGNATURE *(professional establishing POC including prof. designation)*

14. FREQ/DURATION *(e.g., 3/Wk. x 4 Wk.)*

I CERTIFY THE NEED FOR THESE SERVICES FURNISHED UNDER THIS PLAN OF TREATMENT AND WHILE UNDER MY CARE   ☐ N/A

15. PHYSICIAN SIGNATURE   16. DATE

17. CERTIFICATION

FROM   THROUGH   N/A

18. ON FILE *(Print/type physician's name)*
☐

20. INITIAL ASSESSMENT *(History, medical complications, level of function at start of care. Reason for referral.)*

19. PRIOR HOSPITALIZATION

FROM   TO   N/A

21. FUNCTIONAL LEVEL *(End of billing period)* PROGRESS REPORT   ☐ CONTINUE SERVICES **OR**   ☐ DC SERVICES

22. SERVICE DATES
FROM   THROUGH

Form CMS-700-(11-91)

INSTRUCTIONS FOR COMPLETION OF FORM CMS-700

(Enter dates as 6 digits, month, day, year)

1. **Patient's Name** - Enter the patient's last name, first name, and middle initial as shown on the health insurance Medicare card.

2. **Provider Number** - Enter the number issued by Medicare to the billing provider *(i.e., 00–7000).*

3. **HICN** - Enter the patient's health insurance number as shown on the health insurance Medicare card, certification award, utilization notice, temporary eligibility notice, or as reported by SSO.

4. **Provider Name** - Enter the name of the Medicare billing provider.

5. **Medical Record No.** - *(optional)* Enter the patient's medical/clinical record number used by the billing provider.

6. **Onset Date** - Enter the date of onset for the patient's primary medical diagnosis, if it is a new diagnosis, or the date of the most recent exacerbation of a previous diagnosis. If the exact date is not known enter 01 for the day *(i.e., 120191).* The date matches occurrence code 11 on the UB-92.

7. **SOC** *(start of care)* **Date** - Enter the date services began at the billing provider (the date of the first Medicare billable visit which **remains the same on subsequent claims** until discharge or denial corresponds to occurrence code 35 for PT, 44 for OT, 45 for SLP, and 46 for CR on the UB-92).

8. **Type** - Check the type therapy billed; i.e., physical therapy (PT), occupational therapy (OT), speech-language pathology (SLP), cardiac rehabilitation (CR), respiratory therapy (RT), psychological services (PS), skilled nursing services (SN), or social services (SW).

9. **Primary Diagnosis** - Enter the pertinent written medical diagnosis resulting in the therapy disorder and relating to 50% or more of effort in the plan of treatment.

10. **Treatment Diagnosis** - Enter the written treatment diagnosis for which services are rendered. For example, for PT the primary medical diagnosis might be Degeneration of Cervical Intervertebral Disc while the PT treatment DX might be Frozen R Shoulder or, for SLP, while CVA might be the primary medical DX, the treatment DX might be Aphasia. If the same as the primary DX enter SAME.

11. **Visits from Start of Care** - Enter the **cumulative total** visits *(sessions)* completed since services were started at the billing provider for the diagnosis treated, through the last visit on this bill. *(Corresponds to UB-92 value code 50 for PT, 51 for OT, 52 for SLP, or 53 for cardiac rehab.)*

12. **Plan of Treatment/Functional Goals** - Enter brief current plan of treatment goals for the patient for this billing period. Enter the major short-term goals to reach overall long-term outcome. Enter the major plan of treatment to reach stated goals and outcome. Estimate time-frames to reach goals, when possible.

13. **Signature** - Enter the signature *(or name)* and the professional designation of the professional establishing the plan of treatment.

14. **Frequency/Duration** - Enter the current frequency and duration of your treatment; e.g., 3 times per week for 4 weeks is entered 3/Wk x 4Wk.

15. **Physician's Signature** - If the form CMS-700 is used for certification, the physician enters his/her signature. **If certification is required and the form is not being used for certification, check the ON FILE box in item 18.** If the certification is not required for the type service rendered, check the N/A box.

16. **Date** - Enter the date of the physician's signature only if the form is used for certification.

17. **Certification** - Enter the inclusive dates of the certification, **even if the ON FILE box is checked in item 18.** Check the N/A box if certification is not required.

18. **ON FILE** (Means certification signature and date) - Enter the **typed/printed name of the physician** who certified the plan of treatment that is on file at the billing provider. If certification is not required for the type of service checked in item 8, type/print the name of the physician who referred or ordered the service, **but do not check the ON FILE box.**

19. **Prior Hospitalization** - Enter the inclusive dates of recent hospitalization *(1st to DC day)* **pertinent** to the patient's current plan of treatment. Enter N/A if the hospital stay does not relate to the rehabilitation being rendered.

20. **Initial Assessment** - Enter only **current relevant history** from records or patient interview. Enter the major functional limitations stated, if possible, in objective measurable terms. Include only relevant surgical procedures, prior hospitalization and/or therapy for the same condition. Include only pertinent baseline tests and measurements from which to judge future progress or lack of progress.

21. **Functional Level** (end of billing period) - Enter the pertinent progress made and functional levels obtained at the end of the billing period compared to levels shown on initial assessment. Use objective terminology. Date progress when function can be consistently performed. When only a few visits have been made, enter a note indicating the training/treatment rendered and the patient's response if there is no change in function.

22. **Service Dates** - Enter the From and Through dates which represent this billing period *(should be monthly).* Match the From and Through dates in field 6 on the UB-92. DO NOT use 00 in the date. Example: 01 08 91 for January 8, 1991.

C

CMS Forms 1450 and 1500 with Instructions

CMS 1450 Form

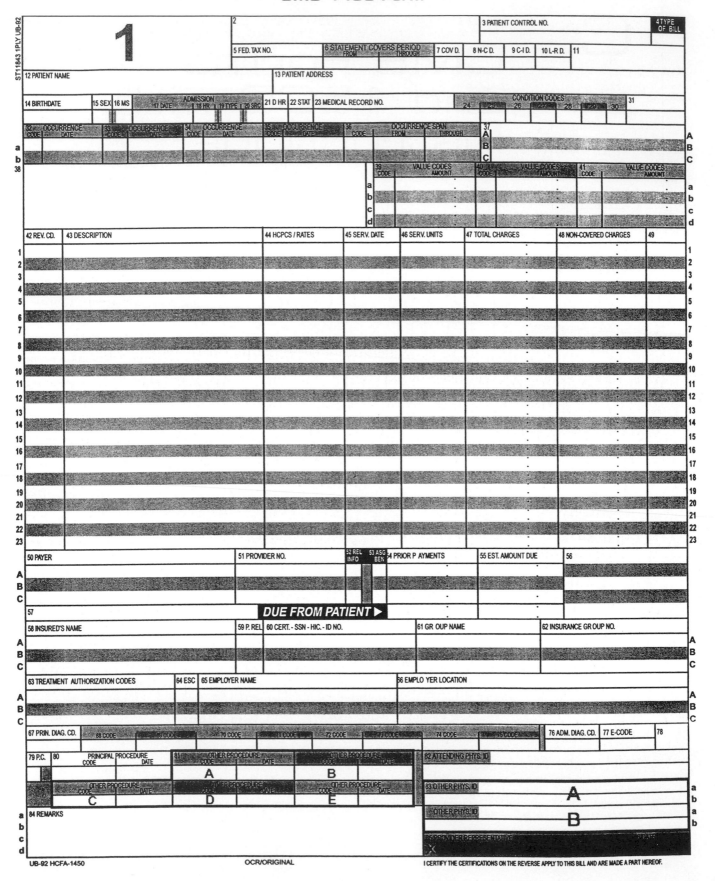

CMS 1450 Form Instructions

UNIFORM BILL: **NOTICE: ANYONE WHO MISREPRESENTS OR FALSIFIES ESSENTIAL INFORMATION REQUESTED BY THIS FORM MAY UPON CONVICTION BE SUBJECT TO FINE AND IMPRISONMENT UNDER FEDERAL AND/OR STATE LAW.**

Certifications relevant to the Bill and Information Shown on the Face Hereof: Signatures on the face hereof incorporate the following certifications or verifications where pertinent to this Bill:

1. If third party benefits are indicated as being assigned or in participation status, on the face thereof, appropriate assignments by the insured beneficiary and signature of patient or parent or legal guardian covering authorization to release information are on file. Determinations as to the release of medical and financial information should be guided by the particular terms of the release forms that were executed by the patient or the patient's legal representative. The hospital agrees to save harmless, indemnify and defend any insurer who makes payment in reliance upon this certification, from and against any claim to the insurance proceeds when in fact no valid assignment of benefits to the hospital was made.

2. If patient occupied a private room or required private nursing for medical necessity, any required certifications are on file.

3. Physician's certifications and re-certifications, if required by contract or Federal regulations, are on file.

4. For Christian Science Sanitoriums, verifications and if necessary re-verifications of the patient's need for sanitorium services are on file.

5. Signature of patient or his/her representative on certifications, authorization to release information, and payment request, as required be Federal law and regulations (42 USC 1935f, 42 CFR 424.36, 10 USC 1071 thru 1086, 32 CFR 199) and, any other applicable contract regulations, is on file.

6. This claim, to the best of my knowledge, is correct and complete and is in conformance with the Civil Rights Act of 1964 as amended. Records adequately disclosing services will be maintained and necessary information will be furnished to such governmental agencies as required by applicable law.

7. For Medicare purposes:

    If the patient has indicated that other health insurance or a state medical assistance agency will pay part of his/her medical expenses and he/she wants information about his/her claim released to them upon their request, necessary authorization is on file. The patient's signature on the provider's request to bill Medicare authorizes any holder of medical and non-medical information, including employment status, and whether the person has employer group health insurance, liability, no-fault, workers' compensation, or other insurance which is responsible to pay for the services for which this Medicare claim is made.

8. For Medicaid purposes:

    This is to certify that the foregoing information is true, accurate, and complete.
    I understand that payment and satisfaction of this claim will be from Federal and State funds, and that any false claims, statements, or documents, or concealment of a material fact, may be prosecuted under applicable Federal or State Laws.

9. For CHAMPUS purposes:

    This is to certify that:

    (a) the information submitted as part of this claim is true, accurate and complete, and, the services shown on this form were medically indicated and necessary for the health of the patient;

    (b) the patient has represented that by a reported residential address outside a military treatment center catchment area he or she does not live within a catchment area of a U.S. military or U.S. Public Health Service medical facility, or if the patient resides within a catchment area of such a facility, a copy of a Non-Availability Statement (DD Form 1251) is on file, or the physician has certified to a medical emergency in any assistance where a copy of a Non-Availability Statement is not on file;

    (c) the patient or the patient's parent or guardian has responded directly to the provider's request to identify all health insurance coverages, and that all such coverages are identified on the face of the claim except those that are exclusively supplemental payments to CHAMPUS-determined benefits;

    (d) the amount billed to CHAMPUS has been billed after all such coverages have been billed and paid, excluding Medicaid, and the amount billed to CHAMPUS is that remaining claimed against CHAMPUS benefits;

    (e) the beneficiary's cost share has not been waived by consent or failure to exercise generally accepted billing and collection efforts; and,

    (f) any hospital-based physician under contract, the cost of whose services are allocated in the charges included in this bill, is not an employee or member of the Uniformed Services. For purposes of this certification, an employee of the Uniformed Services is an employee, appointed in civil service (refer to 5 USC 2105), including part-time or intermittent but excluding contract surgeons or other personnel employed by the Uniformed Services through personal service contracts. Similarly, member of the Uniformed Services does not apply to reserve members of the Uniformed Services not on active duty.

    (g) based on the Consolidated Omnibus Budget Reconciliation Act of 1986, all providers participating in Medicare must also participate in CHAMPUS for inpatient hospital services provided pursuant to admissions to hospitals occurring on or after January 1, 1987.

    (h) if CHAMPUS benefits are to be paid in a participating status, I agree to submit this claim to the appropriate CHAMPUS claims processor as a participating provider. I agree to accept the CHAMPUS-determined reasonable charge as the total charge for the medical services or supplies listed on the claim form. I will accept the CHAMPUS-determined reasonable charge even if it is less than the billed amount, and also agree to accept the amount paid by CHAMPUS, combined with the cost-share amount and deductible amount, if any, paid by or on behalf of the patient as full payment for the listed medical services or supplies. I will make no attempt to collect from the patient (or his or her parent or guardian) amounts over the CHAMPUS-determined reasonable charge. CHAMPUS will make any benefits payable directly to me, if I submit this claim as a participating provider.

ESTIMATED CONTRACT BENEFITS

CMS 1500 Form

PLEASE
DO NOT
STAPLE
IN THIS
AREA

CARRIER →

| | PICA | | | | | | | | **HEALTH INSURANCE CLAIM FORM** | | PICA | |

1. MEDICARE   MEDICAID   CHAMPUS   CHAMPVA   GROUP HEALTH PLAN   FECA BLK LUNG   OTHER   **1a.** INSURED'S I.D. NUMBER   (FOR PROGRAM IN ITEM 1)

(Medicare #)   (Medicaid #)   (Sponsor's SSN)   (VA File #)   (SSN or ID)   (SSN)   (ID)

2. PATIENT'S NAME (Last Name, First Name, Middle Initial)   **3.** PATIENT'S BIRTH DATE   MM   DD   YY   SEX   M   F   **4.** INSURED'S NAME (Last Name, First Name, Middle Initial)

5. PATIENT'S ADDRESS (No., Street)   **6.** PATIENT RELATIONSHIP TO INSURED   Self   Spouse   Child   Other   **7.** INSURED'S ADDRESS (No., Street)

CITY   STATE   **8.** PATIENT STATUS   Single   Married   Other   CITY   STATE

ZIP CODE   TELEPHONE (Include Area Code)   ( )   Employed   Full-Time Student   Part-Time Student   ZIP CODE   TELEPHONE (INCLUDE AREA CODE)   ( )

9. OTHER INSURED'S NAME (Last Name, First Name, Middle Initial)   **10.** IS PATIENT'S CONDITION RELATED TO: **11.** INSURED'S POLICY GROUP OR FECA NUMBER

a. OTHER INSURED'S POLICY OR GROUP NUMBER   **a.** EMPLOYMENT? (CURRENT OR PREVIOUS)   YES   NO   **a.** INSURED'S DATE OF BIRTH   MM   DD   YY   SEX   M   F

b. OTHER INSURED'S DATE OF BIRTH   MM   DD   YY   SEX   M   F   **b.** AUTO ACCIDENT?   PLACE (State)   YES   NO   **b.** EMPLOYER'S NAME OR SCHOOL NAME

c. EMPLOYER'S NAME OR SCHOOL NAME   **c.** OTHER ACCIDENT?   YES   NO   **c.** INSURANCE PLAN NAME OR PROGRAM NAME

d. INSURANCE PLAN NAME OR PROGRAM NAME   **10d.** RESERVED FOR LOCAL USE   **d.** IS THERE ANOTHER HEALTH BENEFIT PLAN?   YES   NO   If yes, return to and complete item 9 a-d.

READ BACK OF FORM BEFORE COMPLETING & SIGNING THIS FORM.
12. PATIENT'S OR AUTHORIZED PERSON'S SIGNATURE I authorize the release of any medical or other information necessary to process this claim. I also request payment of government benefits either to myself or to the party who accepts assignment below.

SIGNED _____ DATE _____

13. INSURED'S OR AUTHORIZED PERSON'S SIGNATURE I authorize payment of medical benefits to the undersigned physician or supplier for services described below.

SIGNED _____

PATIENT AND INSURED INFORMATION

14. DATE OF CURRENT: MM   DD   YY   ILLNESS (First symptom) OR INJURY (Accident) OR PREGNANCY(LMP)   **15.** IF PATIENT HAS HAD SAME OR SIMILAR ILLNESS. GIVE FIRST DATE   MM   DD   YY   **16.** DATES PATIENT UNABLE TO WORK IN CURRENT OCCUPATION   FROM   MM   DD   YY   TO   MM   DD   YY

17. NAME OF REFERRING PHYSICIAN OR OTHER SOURCE   **17a.** I.D. NUMBER OF REFERRING PHYSICIAN   **18.** HOSPITALIZATION DATES RELATED TO CURRENT SERVICES   FROM   MM   DD   YY   TO   MM   DD   YY

19. RESERVED FOR LOCAL USE   **20.** OUTSIDE LAB?   YES   NO $ CHARGES

21. DIAGNOSIS OR NATURE OF ILLNESS OR INJURY. (RELATE ITEMS 1,2,3 OR 4 TO ITEM 24E BY LINE)

1. _____ . ___   3. _____ . ___

2. _____ . ___   4. _____ . ___

22. MEDICAID RESUBMISSION CODE   ORIGINAL REF. NO.

23. PRIOR AUTHORIZATION NUMBER

24. A DATE(S) OF SERVICE					B Place of Service	C Type of Service	D PROCEDURES, SERVICES, OR SUPPLIES (Explain Unusual Circumstances) CPT/HCPCS MODIFIER	E DIAGNOSIS CODE	F $ CHARGES	G DAYS OR UNITS	H EPSDT Family Plan	I EMG	J COB	K RESERVED FOR LOCAL USE
From MM	DD	YY	To MM	DD	YY										
1														
2														
3														
4														
5														
6														

25. FEDERAL TAX I.D. NUMBER   SSN   EIN   **26.** PATIENT'S ACCOUNT NO.   **27.** ACCEPT ASSIGNMENT? (For govt. claims, see back)   YES   NO   **28.** TOTAL CHARGE $ **29.** AMOUNT PAID $ **30.** BALANCE DUE $

31. SIGNATURE OF PHYSICIAN OR SUPPLIER INCLUDING DEGREES OR CREDENTIALS (I certify that the statements on the reverse apply to this bill and are made a part thereof.)

SIGNED _____ DATE _____

32. NAME AND ADDRESS OF FACILITY WHERE SERVICES WERE RENDERED (If other than home or office)

33. PHYSICIAN'S, SUPPLIER'S BILLING NAME, ADDRESS, ZIP CODE & PHONE #

PIN# _____ GRP# _____

PHYSICIAN OR SUPPLIER INFORMATION

(APPROVED BY AMA COUNCIL ON MEDICAL SERVICE 8/88)   **PLEASE PRINT OR TYPE**   APPROVED OMB-0938-0008 FORM CMS-1500 (12-90), FORM RRB-1500, APPROVED OMB-1215-0055 FORM OWCP-1500, APPROVED OMB-0720-0001 (CHAMPUS)

CMS 1500 Form Instructions

BECAUSE THIS FORM IS USED BY VARIOUS GOVERNMENT AND PRIVATE HEALTH PROGRAMS, SEE SEPARATE INSTRUCTIONS ISSUED BY APPLICABLE PROGRAMS.

NOTICE: Any person who knowingly files a statement of claim containing any misrepresentation or any false, incomplete or misleading information may be guilty of a criminal act punishable under law and may be subject to civil penalties.

REFERS TO GOVERNMENT PROGRAMS ONLY

MEDICARE AND CHAMPUS PAYMENTS: A patient's signature requests that payment be made and authorizes release of any information necessary to process the claim and certifies that the information provided in Blocks 1 through 12 is true, accurate and complete. In the case of a Medicare claim, the patient's signature authorizes any entity to release to Medicare medical and nonmedical information, including employment status, and whether the person has employ in group health insurance, liability, no-fault, worker's compensation or other insurance which is responsible to pay for the services for which the Medicare claim is made. See 42 CFR 411.24(a). If item 9 is completed, the patient's signature authorizes release of the information to the health plan or agency shown. In Medicare assigned or CHAMPUS participation cases, the physician agrees to accept the charge determination of the Medicare carrier or CHAMPUS fiscal intermediary as the full charge, and the patient is responsible only for the deductible, coinsurance and noncovered services. Coinsurance and the deductible are based upon the charge determination of the Medicare carrier or CHAMPUS fiscal intermediary if this is less than the charge submitted. CHAMPUS is not a health insurance program but makes payment for health benefits provided through certain affiliations with the Uniformed Services. Information on the patient's sponsor should be provided in those items captioned in "Insured"; i.e., items 1a, 4, 6, 7, 9, and 11.

BLACK LUNG AND FECA CLAIMS

The provider agrees to accept the amount paid by the Government as payment in full. See Black Lung and FECA instructions regarding required procedure and diagnosis coding systems.

SIGNATURE OF PHYSICIAN OR SUPPLIER (MEDICARE, CHAMPUS, FECA AND BLACK LUNG)

I certify that the services shown on this form were medically indicated and necessary for the health of the patient and were personally furnished by me or were furnished incident to my professional service by my employee under my immediate personal supervision, except as otherwise expressly permitted by Medicare or CHAMPUS regulations.

For services to be considered as "incident" to a physician's professional service, 1) they must be rendered under the physician's immediate personal supervision by his/her employee, 2) they must be an integral, although incidental part of a covered physician's service, 3) they must be of kinds commonly furnished in physician's offices, and 4) the services of nonphysicians must be included on the physician's bills.

For CHAMPUS claims, I further certify that I (or any employee) who rendered services am not an active duty member of the Uniformed Services or a civilian employee of the United States Government or a contract employee of the United States Government, either civilian or military (refer to 5 USC 5536). For Black-Lung claims, I further certify that the services performed were for a Black Lung-related disorder.

No Part B Medicare benefits may be paid unless this form is received as required by existing law and regulations (42 CFR 424.32).

NOTICE: Any one who misrepresents or falsifies essential information to receive payment from Federal funds requested by this form may upon conviction be subject to fine and imprisonment under applicable Federal laws.

NOTICE TO PATIENT ABOUT THE COLLECTION AND USE OF MEDICARE, CHAMPUS, FECA, AND BLACK LUNG INFORMATION
(PRIVACY ACT STATEMENT)

We are authorized by CMS, CHAMPUS and OWCP to ask you for information needed in the administration of the Medicare, CHAMPUS, FECA, and Black Lung programs. Authority to collect information is in section 205(a), 1862, 1872 and 1874 of the Social Security Act as amended, 42 CFR 411.24(a) and 424.5(a) (6), and 44 USC 3101;41 CFR 101 et seq and 10 USC 1079 and 1086; 5 USC 8101 et seq; and 30 USC 901 et seq; 38 USC 613; E.O. 9397.

The information we obtain to complete claims under these programs is used to identify you and to determine your eligibility. It is also used to decide if the services and supplies you received are covered by these programs and to insure that proper payment is made.

The information may also be given to other providers of services, carriers, intermediaries, medical review boards, health plans, and other organizations or Federal agencies, for the effective administration of Federal provisions that require other third parties payers to pay primary to Federal program, and as otherwise necessary to administer these programs. For example, it may be necessary to disclose information about the benefits you have used to a hospital or doctor. Additional disclosures are made through routine uses for information contained in systems of records.

FOR MEDICARE CLAIMS: See the notice modifying system No. 09-70-0501, titled, 'Carrier Medicare Claims Record,' published in the Federal Register, Vol. 55 No. 177, page 37549, Wed. Sept. 12, 1990, or as updated and republished.

FOR OWCP CLAIMS: Department of Labor, Privacy Act of 1974, "Republication of Notice of Systems of Records," Federal Register Vol. 55 No. 40, Wed Feb. 28, 1990, See ESA-5, ESA-6, ESA-12, ESA-13, ESA-30, or as updated and republished.

FOR CHAMPUS CLAIMS: PRINCIPLE PURPOSE(S): To evaluate eligibility for medical care provided by civilian sources and to issue payment upon establishment of eligibility and determination that the services/supplies received are authorized by law.

ROUTINE USE(S): Information from claims and related documents may be given to the Dept. of Veterans Affairs, the Dept. of Health and Human Services and/or the Dept. of Transportation consistent with their statutory administrative responsibilities under CHAMPUS/CHAMPVA; to the Dept. of Justice for representation of the Secretary of Defense in civil actions; to the Internal Revenue Service, private collection agencies, and consumer reporting agencies in connection with recoupment claims; and to Congressional Offices in response to inquiries made at the request of the person to whom a record pertains. Appropriate disclosures may be made to other federal, state, local, foreign government agencies, private business entities, and individual providers of care, on matters relating to entitlement, claims adjudication, fraud, program abuse, utilization review, quality assurance, peer review, program integrity, third-party liability, coordination of benefits, and civil and criminal litigation related to the operation of CHAMPUS.

DISCLOSURES: Voluntary; however, failure to provide information will result in delay in payment or may result in denial of claim. With the one exception discussed below, there are no penalties under these programs for refusing to supply information. However, failure to furnish information regarding the medical services rendered or the amount charged would prevent payment of claims under these programs. Failure to furnish any other information, such as name or claim number, would delay payment of the claim. Failure to provide medical information under FECA could be deemed an obstruction.

It is mandatory that you tell us if you know that another party is responsible for paying for your treatment. Section 1128B of the Social Security Act and 31 USC 3801-3812 provide penalties for withholding this information.

You should be aware that P.L. 100-503, the "Computer Matching and Privacy Protection Act of 1988", permits the government to verify information by way of computer matches.

MEDICAID PAYMENTS (PROVIDER CERTIFICATION)

I hereby agree to keep such records as are necessary to disclose fully the extent of services provided to individuals under the State's Title XIX plan and to furnish information regarding any payments claimed for providing such services as the State Agency or Dept. of Health and Humans Services may request.

I further agree to accept, as payment in full, the amount paid by the Medicaid program for those claims submitted for payment under that program, with the exception of authorized deductible, coinsurance, co-payment or similar cost-sharing charge.

SIGNATURE OF PHYSICIAN (OR SUPPLIER): I certify that the services listed above were medically indicated and necessary to the health of this patient and were personally furnished by me or my employee under my personal direction.

NOTICE: This is to certify that the foregoing information is true, accurate and complete. I understand that payment and satisfaction of this claim will be from Federal and State funds, and that any false claims, statements, or documents, or concealment of a material fact, may be prosecuted under applicable Federal or State laws.

According to the Paperwork Reduction Act of 1995, no persons are required to respond to a collection of information unless it displays a valid OMB control number. The valid OMB control number for this information collection is 0938-0008. The time required to complete this information collection is estimated to average 10 minutes per response, including the time to review instructions, search existing data resources, gather the data needed, and complete and review the information collection. If you have any comments concerning the accuracy of the time estimate(s) or suggestions for improving this form, please write to: CMS, N2-14-26, 7500 Security Boulevard, Baltimore, Maryland 21244-1850.

ICD-9 Code Terms

ICD-9 Codes That Support Medical Necessity (not an inclusive list) for billing purposes, the following diagnoses usually describe an acute event or a complex medical condition that is generally considered acceptable.

138	Late effects of acute poliomyelitis
274.0	Gouty arthropathy
332.0–332.1	Parkinson's disease
333.0	Other degenerative diseases of the basal ganglia
333.6	Idiopathic torsion dystonia
333.7	Symptomatic torsion dystonia
333.83	Spasmodic torticollis
333.84	Organic writers' cramp
333.91	Stiff-man syndrome
334.0–334.8	Spinocerebellar disease
335.0–335.8	Anterior horn cell disease
336.0–336.8	Other diseases of spinal cord
337.20–337.29	Reflex sympathetic dystrophy
340	Multiple sclerosis
341.1	Schilder's disease
341.8	Other demyelinating diseases of central nervous system
342.00–342.92	Hemiplegia and hemiparesis
343.0–343.8	Infantile cerebral palsy
344.00–344.89	Other paralytic syndromes
353.0–353.8	Nerve root and plexus disorders
354.0–354.8	Mononeuritis of upper limb and mononeuritis multiplex
355.0–355.79	Mononeuritis of lower limb
356.0–356.8	Hereditary and idiopathic peripheral neuropathy
357.0–357.8	Inflammatory and toxic neuropathy
358.0–358.8	Myoneural disorders
359.0–359.8	Muscular dystrophies and other myopathies
430	Subarachnoid hemorrhage
431	Intracerebral hemorrhage
432.0	Nontraumatic extradural hemorrhage
432.1	Subdural hemorrhage
436	Acute, but ill-defined, cerebrovascular disease
438.0–438.89	Late effects of cerebrovascular disease
440.23	Atherosclerosis of native arteries of extremities with ulceration
440.24	Atherosclerosis of native arteries of extremities with gangrene
454.0–454.2	Varicose veins of lower extremities
457.0	Postmastectomy lymphedema syndrome
457.1	Other lymphedema
681.00–681.11	Cellulitis and abscess of finger and toe

682.3–682.7	Other cellulitis and abscess
695.81–695.89	Other specified erythematous conditions
696.0	Psoriatic arthropathy
696.1	Other psoriasis
707.0–707.8	Chronic ulcer of skin
709.2	Scar conditions and fibrosis of skin
710.1	Systemic sclerosis
710.3	Dermatomyositis
710.4	Polymyositis
710.8	Other specified diffuse diseases of connective tissue
711.00–711.99	Arthropathy associated with infections
712.10–712.99	Crystal arthropathies
713.0–713.8	Arthropathy associated with other disorders classified elsewhere
714.0–714.9	Rheumatoid arthritis and other inflammatory polyarthropathies
715.00–715.98	Osteoarthrosis and allied disorders
716.00–716.99	Other and unspecified arthropathies
717.0–717.43	Internal derangement of knee
718.00–718.89	Other derangement of joint
719.00–719.89	Other disorders of joint
720.0–720.9	Ankylosing spondylitis and other inflammatory spondylopathies
721.0–721.91	Spondylosis and allied disorders
722.0–722.93	Intervertebral disc disorders
723.0–723.9	Other disorders of cervical region
724.0–724.8	Other disorders of back
725	Polymyalgia rheumatica
726.0–726.91	Peripheral enthesopathies and allied syndromes
727.00–727.89	Other disorders of synovium, tendon, and bursa
728.0–728.89	Disorders of muscle, ligament, and fascia
729.0–729.9	Other disorders of soft tissues
733.10–733.19	Pathologic fracture
754.1	Certain congenital musculoskeletal deformities of sternocleidomastoid muscle
755.30–755.39	Reduction deformities of lower limb
755.60–755.64	Other anomalies of lower limb, including pelvic girdle
781.0	Abnormal involuntary movements
781.2	Abnormality of gait
781.3	Lack of coordination
781.4	Transient paralysis of limb
781.8	Neurologic neglect syndrome
782.3	Edema
799.4	Cachexia
805.00–805.9	Fracture of vertebral column without mention of spinal cord injury
806.00–806.9	Fracture of vertebral column with spinal cord injury
807.00–807.4	Fracture of rib(s) and sternum
808.0–808.9	Fracture of pelvis
809.0–809.1	Ill-defined fractures of bones of trunk
810.00–810.13	Fracture of clavicle
811.00–811.19	Fracture of scapula
812.00–812.59	Fracture of humerus
813.00–813.93	Fracture of radius and ulna
814.00–814.19	Fracture of carpal bone(s)
815.00–815.19	Fracture of metacarpal bone(s)

816.00–816.13	Fracture of one or more phalanges of hand
817.0–817.1	Multiple fractures of hand bones
818.0–818.1	Ill-defined fractures of upper limb
820.00–820.9	Fracture of neck of femur
821.00–821.39	Fracture of other and unspecified parts of femur
822.0–822.1	Fracture of patella
823.00–823.92	Fracture of tibia and fibula
824.0–824.9	Fracture of ankle
825.0–825.39	Fracture of one or more tarsal and metatarsal bones
826.0–826.1	Fracture of one or more phalanges of foot
827.0–827.1	Other, multiple, and ill-defined fractures of lower limb
831.00–831.19	Dislocation of shoulder
832.00–832.19	Dislocation of elbow
833.00–833.19	Dislocation of wrist
834.00–834.12	Dislocation of finger
835.00–835.13	Dislocation of hip
836.0–836.69	Dislocation of knee
837.0–837.1	Dislocation of ankle
838.00–838.19	Dislocation of foot
840.0–840.9	Sprains and strains of shoulder and upper arm
841.0–841.9	Sprains and strains of elbow and forearm
842.00–842.19	Sprains and strains of wrist and hand
843.0–843.9	Sprains and strains of hip and thigh
844.0–844.9	Sprains and strains of knee and leg
845.00–845.19	Sprains and strains of ankle and foot
846.0–846.9	Sprains and strains of sacroiliac region
847.0–847.9	Sprains and strains of other and unspecified parts of back
880.00–880.29	Open wound of shoulder and upper arm
881.00–881.22	Open wound of elbow, forearm, and wrist
882.0–882.2	Open wound of hand except finger(s) alone
883.0–883.2	Open wound of finger(s)
884.0–884.2	Multiple and unspecified open wound of upper limb
885.0–885.1	Traumatic amputation of thumb (complete) (partial)
886.0–886.1	Traumatic amputation of other finger(s) (complete) (partial)
887.0–887.7	Traumatic amputation of arm and hand (complete) (partial)
890.0–890.2	Open wound of hip and thigh
891.0–891.2	Open wound of knee, leg (except thigh), and ankle
892.0–892.2	Open wound of foot except toe(s) alone
893.0–893.2	Open wound of toe(s)
896.0–896.3	Traumatic amputation of foot (complete) (partial)
897.0–897.7	Traumatic amputation of leg(s) (complete) (partial)
905.1–905.9	Late effects of musculoskeletal and connective tissue injuries
923.00–923.9	Contusion of upper limb
924.00–924.4	Contusion of lower limb
926.0–926.8	Crushing injury of trunk
927.00–927.8	Crushing injury of upper limb
928.00–928.8	Crushing injury of lower limb
929.0	Crushing injury of multiple sites, not elsewhere classified
942.20–942.59	Burn of trunk
943.20–943.59	Burn of upper limb, except wrist and hand
944.20–944.58	Burn of wrist(s) and hand(s)
945.20–945.59	Burn of lower limb(s)
946.2–946.5	Burns of multiple specified sites
948.00–948.99	Burns classified according to extent of body surface involved

951.4	Injury to facial nerve
952.00–952.9	Spinal cord injury without evidence of spinal bone injury
953.0–953.8	Injury to nerve roots and spinal plexus
955.0–955.9	Injury to peripheral nerve(s) of shoulder girdle and upper limb
956.0–956.9	Injury to peripheral nerve(s) of pelvic girdle and lower limb
997.61–997.62	Amputation stump complication
V43.61–V43.69	Organ or tissue replaced by joint
V43.7	Organ or tissue replaced by limb
V49.1–V49.77	Problems with limbs and other problems
V52.0	Fitting and adjustment of artificial arm (complete) (partial)
V52.1	Fitting and adjustment of artificial leg (complete) (partial)
V53.7	Fitting and adjustment of orthopedic devices
V54.0–V54.8	Other orthopedic aftercare

E

APTA Guidelines for Physical Therapy Documentation

Preamble

The American Physical Therapy Association (APTA) is committed to meeting the physical therapy needs of society, to meeting the needs and interests of its members, and to developing and improving the art and science of physical therapy, including practice, education and research. To help meet these responsibilities, the APTA Board of Directors has approved the following guidelines for physical therapy documentation. It is recognized that these guidelines do not reflect all of the unique documentation requirements associated with the many specialty areas within the physical therapy profession. Applicable for both hand written and electronic documentation systems, these guidelines are intended to be used as a foundation for the development of more specific documentation guidelines in specialty areas, while at the same time providing guidance for the physical therapy profession across all practice settings.

It is the position of the American Physical Therapy Association (APTA) that physical therapist examination, evaluation, diagnosis, and prognosis shall be documented, dated, and authenticated by the physical therapist who performs the service. Intervention provided by the physical therapist or physical therapist assistant, under the direction and supervision of a physical therapist, is documented, dated, and authenticated by the physical therapist or, when permissible by law, the physical therapist assistant.

Other notations or flow charts are considered a component of the documented record but do not meet the requirements of documentation in, or of, themselves, *Position on Authority for Physical Therapy Documentation* (HOD 06-00-20-05).

Operational Definitions

Guidelines: APTA defines "guidelines" as approved, non-binding statements of advice. Documentation: Any entry into the client record, such as: consultation report, initial examination report, progress note, flow sheet/checklist that identifies the care/service provided, re-examination, or summation of care.

Authentication: The process used to verify that an entry is complete, accurate and final. Indications of authentication can include original written signatures and computer "signatures" on secured electronic record systems only.

I. General Guidelines

All documentation must comply with the applicable jurisdictional/regulatory requirements.

1. All handwritten entries shall be made in ink and will include original signatures. Electronic entries are made with appropriate security and confidentiality provisions.

2. Charting errors should be corrected by drawing a single line through the error and initialing and dating the chart or through the appropriate mechanism for electronic documentation that clearly indicates that a change was made without deletion of the original record.

3. Identification.

    3.1 Include patient/client's full name and identification number, if applicable, on all official documents.

    3.2 All entries must be dated and authenticated with the provider's full name and appropriate designation, i.e., PT or PTA.

    3.3 Documentation by graduates or others pending receipt of an unrestricted license shall be authenticated by a licensed physical therapist.

    3.4 Documentation by students (SPT/SPTA) in physical therapist or physical therapist assistant programs must be additionally authenticated by the physical therapist or, when permissible by law, documentation by physical therapist assistant students may be authenticated by a physical therapist assistant.

4. Documentation should include the referral mechanism by which physical therapy services are initiated:

    Examples include:

        Ex 4.1: Self-referral/direct access

        Ex 4.2: Request for consultation from another practitioner

II. Initial Patient/Client Management

A. Documentation is required at the onset of each episode of physical therapy care and shall include the elements of examination, evaluation, diagnosis, and prognosis.

B. Documentation of the initial episode of physical therapy care shall include the elements of examination, a comprehensive screening and specific testing process leading to diagnostic classification, or, as appropriate, to a referral to another practitioner. The examination has three components: the patient/client history, the systems review, and tests and measures.

1. Documentation of appropriate history:

    1.1 General demographics

        Social history

        Employment/work (Job/School/Play)

        Growth and development

        Living environment

        General health status (self-report, family report, caregiver report)

        Social/health habits (past and current)

        Family history

        Medical/surgical history

        Current condition(s)/Chief complaint(s)

        Functional status and activity level

        Medications

        Other clinical tests

2. Documentation of systems review

2.1 Documentation of physiologic and anatomical status to include the following systems:

Cardiovascular/pulmonary

Blood Pressure

Edema

Heart Rate

Respiratory Rate

Integumentary

Presence of scar formation

Skin color

Skin integrity

Musculoskeletal

Gross range of motion

Gross strength

Gross symmetry

Height

Weight

Neuromuscular

Gross coordinated movement (e.g., balance, locomotion, transfers, and transitions)

2.2 A review of communication ability, affect, cognition, language, and learning style

Ability to make needs known

Consciousness

Orientation

Expected emotional/behavioral responses

Learning preferences

3. Documentation of selection and administration of appropriate tests and measures to determine patient/client status in a number of areas and documentation of findings. The following is a list of the areas that may be addressed in the documented examination and evaluation, including categories of tests and measures for each area:

Aerobic Capacity/Endurance

Examples of examination findings include:

Ex 3.1.1   Aerobic capacity during functional activities

Ex 3.1.2   Aerobic capacity during standardized exercise test protocols

Ex 3.1.3   Cardiovascular signs and symptoms in response to increased oxygen demand with exercise or activity

Ex 3.1.4   Pulmonary signs and symptoms in response to increased oxygen demand with exercise or activity

Anthropometric Characteristics

Examples of examination findings include:

Ex 3.2.1   Body composition

Ex 3.2.2   Body dimensions

Ex 3.2.3   Edema

Arousal, Attention, and Cognition

Examples of examination findings include:

Ex 3.3.1   Arousal and attention

Ex 3.3.2   Cognition

Ex 3.3.3   Communication

Ex 3.3.4   Consciousness

Ex 3.3.5   Motivation

Ex 3.3.6   Orientation to time, person, place, and situation

Ex 3.3.7   Recall

Assistive and Adaptive Devices

Examples of examination findings include:

Ex 3.4.1   Assistive or adaptive devices and equipment use during functional activities

Ex 3.4.2   Components, alignment, fit, and ability to care for the assistive or adaptive devices and equipment

Ex 3.4.3   Remediation of impairments, functional limitations, or disabilities with use of assistive or adaptive devices and equipment

Ex 3.4.4   Safety during use of assistive or adaptive devices and equipment

Circulation (Arterial, Venous, Lymphatic)

Examples of examination findings include:

Ex 3.5.2   Cardiovascular symptoms

Ex 3.5.3   Physiological responses to position change

Cranial and Peripheral Nerve Integrity

Examples of examination findings include:

Ex 3.6.1   Electrophysiological integrity

Ex 3.6.2   Motor distribution of the cranial nerves

Ex 3.6.3   Motor distribution of the peripheral nerves

Ex 3.6.4   Response to neural provocation

Ex 3.6.5   Response to stimuli, including auditory, gustatory, olfactory, pharyngeal, vestibular, and visual

Ex 3.6.6   Sensory distribution of the cranial nerves

Ex 3.6.7   Sensory distribution of the peripheral nerves

Environmental, Home, and Work (Job/School/Play) Barriers

Examples of examination findings include:

Ex 3.7.1   Current and potential barriers

Ex 3.7.2   Physical space and environment

Ergonomics and Body Mechanics

Examples of examination findings for ergonomics include:

Ex 3.8.1   Dexterity and coordination during work

Ex 3.8.2   Functional capacity and performance during work actions, tasks, or activities

Ex 3.8.3   Safety in work environments

Ex 3.8.4   Specific work conditions or activities

Ex 3.8.5   Tools, devices, equipment, and work-stations related to work actions, tasks, or activities

Examples of examination findings for body mechanics include:

Ex 3.8.6   Body mechanics during self-care, home management, work, community, or leisure actions, tasks, or activities

Gait, Locomotion, and Balance

Examples of examination findings include:

Ex 3.9.1   Balance during functional activities with or without the use of assistive, adaptive, orthotic, protection, supportive, or prosthetic devices or equipment

Ex 3.9.2   Balance (dynamic and static) with or without the use of assistive, adaptive, orthotic, protective, supportive, or prosthetic devices or equipment

Ex 3.9.3   Gait and locomotion during functional activities with or without the use of assistive, adaptive, orthotic, protective, supportive, or prosthetic devices or equipment

Ex 3.9.4   Gait and locomotion with or without the use of assistive, adaptive, orthotic, protective, supportive, or prosthetic devices or equipment

Ex 3.9.5   Safety during gait, locomotion, and balance

Integumentary Integrity

Examples of examination findings include:

Ex 3.10.1   Associated with skin:

Ex 3.10.1.1   Activities, positioning, and postures that produce or relieve trauma to the skin

Ex 3.10.1.2   Assistive, adaptive, orthotic, protective, supportive, or prosthetic devices and equipment that may produce or relieve trauma to the skin

Ex 3.10.1.3   Skin characteristics

Ex 3.10.2   Wound:

Ex 3.10.2.1   Activities, positioning, and postures that aggravate the wound or scar or that produce or relieve trauma

Ex 3.10.2.2   Burn

Ex 3.10.2.3   Signs of infection

Ex 3.10.2.4   Wound characteristics

Ex 3.10.2.5   Wound scar tissue characteristics

Joint Integrity

Examples of examination findings include:

Ex 3.11.1   Joint integrity and mobility

Ex 3.11.2   Joint play movements

Ex 3.11.3   Specific body parts

Motor Function

Examples of examination findings include:

Ex 3.12.1   Dexterity, coordination, and agility

Ex 3.12.2   Electrophysiological integrity

Ex 3.12.3   Hand function

Ex 3.12.4   Initiation, modification, and control of movement patterns and voluntary postures

Muscle Performance

Examples of examination findings include:

Ex 3.13.1   Electrophysiological integrity

Ex 3.13.2   Muscle strength, power, and endurance

Ex 3.13.3   Muscle strength, power, and endurance during functional activities

Ex 3.13.4   Muscle tension

Neuromotor Development and Sensory Integration

Examples of examination findings include:

Ex 3.14.1   Acquisition and evolution of motor skills

Ex 3.14.2   Oral motor function, phonation, and speech production

Ex 3.14.3   Sensorimotor integration

Orthotic, Protective, and Supportive Devices

Examples of examination findings include:

Ex 3.15.1   Components, alignment, fit, and ability to care for the orthotic, protective, and supportive devices and equipment

Ex 3.15.2   Orthotic, protective, and supportive devices and equipment use during functional activities

Ex 3.15.3   Remediation of impairments, functional limitations, or disabilities with use of orthotic, protective, and supportive devices and equipment

Ex 3.15.4   Safety during use of orthotic, protective, and supportive devices and equipment

Pain

Examples of examination findings include:

Ex 3.16.1   Pain, soreness, and nociception

Ex 3.16.2   Pain in specific body parts

Posture

Examples of examination findings include:

Ex 3.17.1   Postural alignment and position (dynamic)

Ex 3.17.2   Postural alignment and position (static)

Ex 3.17.3   Specific body parts

Prosthetic Requirements

Examples of examination findings include:

Ex 3.18.1   Components, alignment, fit, and ability to care for prosthetic device

Ex 3.18.2   Prosthetic device use during functional activities

Ex 3.18.3   Remediation of impairments, functional limitations, or disabilities with use of the prosthetic device

Ex 3.18.4   Residual limb or adjacent segment

Ex 3.18.5   Safety during use of the prosthetic device

Range of Motion (Including Muscle Length)

Examples of examination findings include:

Ex 3.19.1   Functional ROM

Ex 3.19.2   Joint active and passive movement

Ex 3.19.3   Muscle length, soft tissue extensibility, and flexibility

Reflex Integrity

Examples of examination findings include:

Ex 3.20.1   Deep reflexes

Ex 3.20.2   Electrophysiological integrity

Ex 3.20.3   Postural reflexes and reactions, including righting, equilibrium, and protective reactions

Ex 3.20.4   Primitive reflexes and reactions

Ex 3.20.5   Resistance to passive stretch

Ex 3.20.6   Superficial reflexes and reactions

Self-Care and Home Management

Examples of examination findings include:

Ex 3.21.1   Ability to gain access to home environments

Ex 3.21.2   Ability to perform self-care and home management activities with or without assistive, adaptive, orthotic, protective, supportive, or prosthetic devices and equipment

Ex 3.21.3   Safety in self-care and home management activities and environments

Sensory Integrity

Examples of examination findings include:

Ex 3.22.1   Combined/cortical sensations

Ex 3.22.2   Deep sensations

Ex 3.22.3   Electrophysiological integrity

Ventilation and Respiration

Examples of examination findings include:

Ex 3.23.1   Pulmonary signs of respiration/gas exchange

Ex 3.23.2   Pulmonary signs of ventilatory function

Ex 3.23.3   Pulmonary symptoms

Ex 3.23.4   Work (job/school/play), community, and leisure integration or reintegration

Examples of examination findings include:

Ex 3.24.1   Ability to assume or resume work (job/school/plan), community, and leisure activities with or without assistive, adaptive, orthotic, protective, supportive, or prosthetic devices and equipment

Ex 3.24.2   Ability to gain access to work (job/school/play), community, and leisure environments

Ex 3.24.3   Safety in work (job/school/play), community, and leisure activities and environments

C. Documentation of evaluation (a dynamic process in which the physical therapist makes clinical judgments based on data gathered during the examination).

D. Documentation of diagnosis (a label encompassing a cluster of signs and symptoms, syndromes, or categories that reflects the information obtained from the examination).

E. Documentation of prognosis (determination of the level of optimal improvement that might be attained through intervention and the amount of time required to reach that level. Documentation shall include anticipated goals, expected outcomes, and plan of care).

1. Patient/client (and family members and significant others, if appropriate) is involved in establishing anticipated goals and expected outcomes.

2. All anticipated goals and expected outcomes are stated in measurable terms.

3. Anticipated goals and expected outcomes are related to impairments, functional limitations, and disabilities and the changes in health, wellness, and fitness needs identified in the examination.

4. The plan of care:

    4.1 Is based on the examination, evaluation, diagnosis, and prognosis

    4.2 Identifies anticipated goals and expected outcomes of all proposed interventions

    4.3 Describes the proposed interventions taking into consideration the expectations of the patient/client and others as appropriate

    4.4 Includes frequency and duration of all proposed interventions to achieve the anticipated goals and expected outcomes

    4.5 Involves appropriate coordination and communication of care with other professionals/services.

    4.6 Includes plan for discharge

F. Authentication by and appropriate designation of the physical therapist.

III. Documentation of the Continuation of Care

A. Documentation of intervention or services provided and current patient/client status.

1. Documentation is required for every visit/encounter.

    1.1 Authentication and appropriate designation of the physical therapist, or the physical therapist assistant providing the service under the direction and supervision of a physical therapist.

2. Documentation of each visit/encounter shall include the following elements:

    2.1 Patient/client self-report (as appropriate).

    2.2 Identification of specific interventions provided, including frequency, intensity, and duration as appropriate.

    Examples include:

    Knee extension, three sets, ten repetitions, 10# weight

    Transfer training bed to chair with sliding board

    2.3 Equipment provided

    2.4 Changes in patient/client status as they relate to the plan of care.

    2.5 Adverse reaction to interventions, if any.

    2.6 Factors that modify frequency or intensity of intervention and progression toward anticipated goals and expected outcomes, including patient/client adherence to patient/client-related instructions.

    2.7 Communication/consultation with providers/patient/client/family/significant other.

B. Documentation of Reexamination

1. Documentation of reexamination provided as appropriate, to evaluate progress and to modify or redirect intervention.

2. Documentation of reexamination shall include the following elements:

    2.1 Documentation of selected components of examination to update patient/client's status.

    2.2 Interpretation of findings and, when indicated, revision of anticipated goals and expected outcomes.

    2.3 When indicated, revision of plan of care, as directly correlated with anticipated goals and expected outcomes as documented.

    2.4 Authentication by and appropriate designation of the physical therapist.

IV. Documentation of Summation of Episode of Care

    A. Documentation is required following conclusion of the current episode in the physical therapy intervention sequence.

    B. Documentation of the summation of the episode of care shall include the following elements:

        1. Criteria for termination of services:

        Examples of discharge include:

        Ex 1.1   Anticipated goals and expected outcomes have been achieved.

        Examples of discontinuation include:

        Ex 1.2   Patient/client, caregiver, or legal guardian declines to continue intervention.

        Ex 1.3   Patient/client is unable to continue to progress toward anticipated goals due to medical or psychosocial complications or because financial/insurance resources have been expended.

        Ex 1.4   Physical therapist determines that the patient/client will no longer benefit from physical therapy.

        2. Current physical/functional status.

        3. Degree of anticipated goals and expected outcomes achieved and reasons for goals and outcomes not being achieved.

        4. Discharge or discontinuation plan that includes written and verbal communication related to the patient/client's continuing care.

        Examples include:

        Ex 4.1   Home program.

        Ex 4.2   Referrals for additional services.

        Ex 4.3   Recommendations for follow-up physical therapy care.

        Ex 4.4   Family and caregiver training.

        Ex 4.5   Equipment provided.

        5. Authentication by and appropriate designation of the physical therapist.

Additional References

1. *Direction and Supervision of the Physical Therapist Assistant* (HOD 06-00-16-27).

2. *Comprehensive Accreditation Manual for Hospitals.* Oakbrook Terrace, Ill: Joint Commission on the Accreditation of Healthcare Organizations.

3. *Glossary of Terms Related to Information Security.* Schaumburg, Ill: Computer-based Patient Record Institute.

4. *Guidelines for Establishing Information Security Policies at Organizations Using Computer-based Patient Records.* Schamburg, Ill: Computer-based Patient Record Institute.

5. *Current Procedural Terminology 2000.* American Medical Association (AMA).

6. *Coding and Payment Guide for the Physical Therapist 2000.* St. Anthony's Publishing and the American Physical Therapy Association.

7. Healthcare Finance Administration (HCFA) (www.hcfa.gov): Minimal Data Set (MDS) Regulations, HCFA/AMA Documentation Guidelines, Home Health Regulations.

8. State Practice Acts (www.fsbpt.org).

BOD 11-01-06-10 (Program 32) [Amended BOD 03-01-16-51; BOD 03-00-22-54; BOD 03-99-14-41; BOD 11-98-19-69; BOD 03-97-27-69; BOD 03-95-23-61; BOD 11-94-33-107; BOD 06-93-09-13; Initial BOD 03-93-21-55]

**DOCUMENTATION TEMPLATE FOR
PHYSICAL THERAPIST PATIENT/CLIENT MANAGEMENT**
Inpatient Form, Page 1

Today's Date: _____
Patient ID#: _____

Inpatient History

American Physical Therapy Association

IDENTIFICATION INFORMATION

1 Name: _____

a Last

b First   c MI   d Jr/Sr

2 Admission Date: Month □□   Day □□   Year □□□□

3 Date of Birth: Month □□   Day □□   Year □□□□

4 Sex: a □ Male   b □ Female

5 Dominant Hand: a □ Right   b □ Left   c □ Unknown

6 Race
a □ American Indian or Alaska Native
b □ Asian
c □ Black or African American
d □ Hispanic or Latino
e □ Native Hawaiian or Other Pacific Islander
f □ White

7 Ethnicity
a □ Hispanic or Latino
b □ Not Hispanic or Latino

8 Language
a □ English understood
b □ Interpreter needed
c □ Primary language: _____

9 Education
a Highest grade completed (Circle one): 1 2 3 4 5 6 7 8 9 10 11 12
b □ Some college/technical school
c □ College graduate
d □ Graduate school/advanced degree

10 Has patient completed an advance directive?   a □ Yes   b □ No

11 Referred by: _____

12 Reasons for referral to physical therapy: _____

SOCIAL HISTORY

13 Cultural/Religious
Any customs or religious beliefs or wishes that might affect care?
_____

14 Lives(d) With

	(1)–Admission	(2)–Expected at Discharge
a Alone	□	□
b Spouse only	□	□
c Spouse and other(s)	□	□
d Child (not spouse)	□	□
e Other relative(s) (not spouse or children)	□	□
f Group setting	□	□
g Personal care attendant	□	□
h Unknown	□	□
i Other	_____	

15 Available Social Supports (family/friends)
0=No 1=Possibly yes 2=Definitely

	Now	Willing/Able Postdischarge
a Emotional support	□	□
b Intermittent physical support with ADLs or IADLs—less than daily	□	□
c Intermittent physical support with ADLs or IADLs—daily	□	□
d Full-time physical support (as needed) with ADLs or IADLs	□	□
e All or most of necessary tranportation	□	□

16 Caregiver Status   Presence of family member/friend willing and able to assist patient/client?   a □ Yes   b □ No

17 EMPLOYMENT/WORK (Job/School/Play)
a □ Working full-time outside of home
b □ Working part-time outside of home
c □ Working full-time from home
d □ Working part-time from home
e □ Homemaker
f □ Student
g □ Retired
h □ Unemployed

i Occupation: _____

LIVING ENVIRONMENT

18 Devices and Equipment (e.g., cane, glasses, hearing aids, walker)
_____
_____
_____
_____
_____
_____

19 Type of Residence

	(1)–Admission	(2)–Expected at Discharge
a Private home	□	□
b Private apartment	□	□
c Rented room	□	□
d Board and care/assisted living/group home	□	□
e Homeless (with or without shelter)	□	□
f Long-term care facility (nursing home)	□	□
g Hospice	□	□
h Unknown	□	□
i Other	_____	

20 Environment

	(1)–Admission	(2)–Expected at Discharge
a Stairs, no railing	□	□
b Stairs, railing	□	□
c Ramps	□	□
d Elevator	□	□
e Uneven terrain	□	□
f Other obstacles:	_____	

21 Past Use of Community Services 0=No 1=Unknown 2=Yes

a Day services/programs	□	f Mental health services	□
b Home health services	□	g Respiratory therapy	□
c Homemaking services	□	h Therapies—PT, OT, SLP	□
d Hospice	□	i Other (eg, volunteer)	□
e Meals on Wheels	□	_____	

22 GENERAL HEALTH STATUS
a Patient/client rates health as:
□ Excellent   □ Good   □ Fair   □ Poor

b Major life changes during past year?   (1) □ Yes   (2) □ No

DOCUMENTATION TEMPLATE FOR PHYSICAL THERAPIST PATIENT/CLIENT MANAGEMENT
Inpatient Form, Page 2

23 SOCIAL/HEALTH HABITS (Past and Current)

a Alcohol

(1) How many days per week does patient/client drink beer, wine, or other alcoholic beverages, on average? _____

(2) If one beer, one glass of wine, or one cocktail equals one drink, how many drinks does patient/client have, on an average day? _____

b Smoking

(1) Currently use tobacco.

(a) ☐ Yes

1. ☐ Cigarettes: # of packs per day _____

2. ☐ Cigars/pipes: # per day _____

(b) ☐ No

(2) Smoked in past?   (a) ☐ Yes Year quit: ☐☐☐☐

(b) ☐ No

c Exercise

(1) Exercises beyond normal daily activities and chores?

(a) ☐ Yes

Describe the exercise: _____

1. On average, how many days per week does patient/client exercise or do physical activity? _____

2. For how many minutes, on an average day? __

(b) ☐ No

24 FAMILY HISTORY

Condition:	Relationship to Patient/Client:	Age at Onset (if known):
a Heart disease	_____	_____
b Hypertension	_____	_____
c Stroke	_____	_____
d Diabetes	_____	_____
e Cancer	_____	_____
f Other: _____	_____	_____
_____	_____	_____

25 PATIENT/CLIENT MEDICAL/SURGICAL HISTORY: _____

_____
_____
_____
_____
_____

26 FUNCTIONAL STATUS/ACTIVITY LEVEL (Check all that apply):

a ☐ Difficulty with locomotion/movement:

(1) ☐ bed mobility

(2) ☐ transfers

(3) ☐ gait (walking)

(a) ☐ on level

(b) ☐ on stairs

(c) ☐ on ramps

(d) ☐ on uneven terrain

b ☐ Difficulty with self-care (such as bathing, dressing, eating, toileting)

c ☐ Difficulty with home management (such as household chores, shopping, driving/transportation)

d ☐ Difficulty with community and work activities/integration

(1) ☐ work/school

(2) ☐ recreation or play activity

27 MEDICATIONS (List): _____

_____
_____
_____
_____
_____
_____
_____
_____
_____

28 OTHER CLINICAL TESTS (List):

	Month	Year	Findings
_____	☐☐	☐☐☐☐	_____
_____	☐☐	☐☐☐☐	_____
_____	☐☐	☐☐☐☐	_____
_____	☐☐	☐☐☐☐	

DOCUMENTATION TEMPLATE FOR PHYSICAL THERAPIST
PATIENT/CLIENT MANAGEMENT
Outpatient Form 1, Page 1

Today's Date: _____
Patient ID#: _____

Outpatient History

1 **Name:**
_____
a Last

_____
b First   c MI   d Jr/Sr

2 **Street Address:** _____

_____
City   State   Zip

3 **Date of Birth:** ☐☐ ☐☐ ☐☐☐☐
Month   Day   Year

4 **Sex:** a ☐ Male   b ☐ Female

5 **Are you:** a ☐ Right-handed   b ☐ Left-handed

6 **Type of Insurance:** a ☐ Insurer _____
b ☐ Workers' Comp   c ☐ Medicare   d ☐ Self-pay   e ☐ Other

7 **Race:**
a ☐ American Indian or Alaska Native
b ☐ Asian
c ☐ Black or African American
d ☐ Hispanic or Latino
e ☐ Native Hawaiian or Other Pacific Islander _____
f ☐ White

8 **Ethnicity:**
a ☐ Hispanic or Latino
b ☐ Not Hispanic or Latino

9 **Language:**
a ☐ English understood
b ☐ Interpreter needed
c ☐ Language you speak most often: _____

10 **Education:**
a Highest grade completed (Circle one): 1 2 3 4 5 6 7 8 9 10 11 12
b ☐ Some college/technical school
c ☐ College graduate
d ☐ Graduate school/advanced degree

SOCIAL HISTORY

11 **Cultural/Religious:** Any customs or religious beliefs or wishes that might affect care?
_____

12 **With whom do you live:**
a ☐ Alone
b ☐ Spouse only
c ☐ Spouse and other(s)
d ☐ Child (not spouse)
e ☐ Other relative(s) (not spouse or children)
f ☐ Group setting
g ☐ Personal care attendant
h ☐ Other:

13 **Have you completed an advance directive?** a ☐ Yes   b ☐ No

14 **Who referred you to the physical therapist:**
_____

15 **Employment/Work (Job/School/Play)**
a ☐ Working full-time outside of home
b ☐ Working part-time outside of home
c ☐ Working full-time from home
d ☐ Working part-time from home
e ☐ Homemaker   f ☐ Student   g ☐ Retired   h ☐ Unemployed
i Occupation: _____

LIVING ENVIRONMENT

16 **Does your home have:**
a ☐ Stairs, no railing
b ☐ Stairs, railing
c ☐ Ramps
d ☐ Elevator
e ☐ Uneven terrain
f ☐ Assistive devices (e.g., bathroom): _____
g ☐ Any obstacles: _____

17 **Do you use:**
a ☐ Cane
b ☐ Walker or rollator
c ☐ Manual wheelchair
d ☐ Motorized wheelchair
e ☐ Glasses, hearing aids
f ☐ Other: _____
_____

18 **Where do you live:**
a ☐ Private home
b ☐ Private apartment
c ☐ Rented room
d ☐ Board and care/assisted living/group home
e ☐ Homeless (with or without shelter)
f ☐ Long-term care facility (nursing home)
g ☐ Hospice
h ☐ Other: _____

19 **GENERAL HEALTH STATUS**
a Please rate your health:
(1) ☐ Excellent   (2) ☐ Good   (3) ☐ Fair   (4) ☐ Poor
b Have you had any major life changes during past year? (e.g., new baby, job change, death of a family member) (1) ☐ Yes   (2) ☐ No

20 **SOCIAL/HEALTH HABITS**
a Smoking
(1) Currently smoke tobacco? (a) ☐ Yes   1. ☐ Cigarettes: # of packs per day __
   2. ☐ Cigars/Pipes: # per day __
(b) ☐ No
(2) Smoked in past? (a) ☐ Yes   Year quit: ☐☐☐☐   (b) ☐ No

b Alcohol
(1) How many days per week do you drink beer, wine, or other alcoholic beverages, on average? ____
(2) If one beer, one glass of wine, or one cocktail equals one drink, how many drinks do you have, on an average day? ___

c Exercise
Do you exercise beyond normal daily activities and chores?
(a) ☐ Yes   Describe the exercise: _____
   1. On average, how many days per week do you exercise or do physical activity? _____
   2. For how many minutes, on an average day? ____
(b) ☐ No

21 **FAMILY HISTORY** (Indicate whether mother, father, brother/sister, aunt/uncle, or grandmother/grandfather, and age of onset if known)
a Heart disease: _____
b Hypertension: _____
c Stroke: _____
d Diabetes: _____
e Cancer: _____
f Psychological: _____
g Arthritis: _____
h Osteoporosis: _____
i Other: _____

DOCUMENTATION TEMPLATE FOR PHYSICAL THERAPIST PATIENT/CLIENT MANAGEMENT
Outpatient Form, Page 2

22 MEDICAL/SURGICAL HISTORY

a Please check if you have ever had:

(1) ☐ Arthritis
(2) ☐ Broken bones/ fractures
(3) ☐ Osteoporosis
(4) ☐ Blood disorders
(5) ☐ Circulation/vascular problems
(6) ☐ Heart problems
(7) ☐ High blood pressure
(8) ☐ Lung problems
(9) ☐ Stroke
(10) ☐ Diabetes/ high blood sugar
(11) ☐ Low blood sugar/ hypoglycemia
(12) ☐ Head injury

(13) ☐ Multiple sclerosis
(14) ☐ Muscular dystrophy
(15) ☐ Parkinson disease
(16) ☐ Seizures/epilepsy
(17) ☐ Allergies
(18) ☐ Developmental or growth problems
(19) ☐ Thyroid problems
(20) ☐ Cancer
(21) ☐ Infectious disease (e.g., tuberculosis, hepatitis)
(22) ☐ Kidney problems
(23) ☐ Repeated infections
(24) ☐ Ulcers/stomach problems
(25) ☐ Skin diseases
(26) ☐ Depression
(27) ☐ Other:_____

b Within the past year, have you had any of the following symptoms? (Check all that apply)

(1) ☐ Chest pain
(2) ☐ Heart palpitations
(3) ☐ Cough
(4) ☐ Hoarseness
(5) ☐ Shortness of breath
(6) ☐ Dizziness or blackouts
(7) ☐ Coordination problems
(8) ☐ Weakness in arms or legs
(9) ☐ Loss of balance
(10) ☐ Difficulty walking
(11) ☐ Joint pain or swelling
(12) ☐ Pain at night

(13) ☐ Difficulty sleeping
(14) ☐ Loss of appetite
(15) ☐ Nausea/vomiting
(16) ☐ Difficulty swallowing
(17) ☐ Bowel problems
(18) ☐ Weight loss/gain
(19) ☐ Urinary problems
(20) ☐ Fever/chills/sweats
(21) ☐ Headaches
(22) ☐ Hearing problems
(23) ☐ Vision problems
(24) ☐ Other:_____

c Have you ever had surgery? (1) ☐ Yes (2) ☐ No
If yes, please describe, and include dates:

Month Year
_____ ☐☐ ☐☐☐☐
_____ ☐☐ ☐☐☐☐
_____ ☐☐ ☐☐☐☐

For men only: d Have you been diagnosed with prostate disease?
(1) ☐ Yes (2) ☐ No

For women only:
Have you been diagnosed with:
e Pelvic inflammatory disease?
(1) ☐ Yes (2) ☐ No
f Endometriosis?
(1) ☐ Yes (2) ☐ No
g Trouble with your period?
(1) ☐ Yes (2) ☐ No

h Complicated pregnancies or deliveries?
(1) ☐ Yes (2) ☐ No
i Pregnant, or think you might be pregnant?
(1) ☐ Yes (2) ☐ No
j Other gynecological or obstetrical difficulties?
(1) ☐ Yes (2) ☐ No
If yes, please describe:_____

23 CURRENT CONDITION(S)/CHIEF COMPLAINT(S)

a Describe the problem(s) for which you seek physical therapy:
_____
_____

Month Year
b When did the problem(s) begin (date)? ☐☐ ☐☐☐☐
c What happened? _____
_____

d Have you ever had the problem(s) before?
(1) ☐ Yes
(a) What did you do for the problem(s)? _____
_____
(b) Did the problem(s) get better?
1. ☐ Yes 2. ☐ No
(c) About how long did the problem(s) last?_____
(2) ☐ No

23 Current Condition(s)/Chief Complaint(s) (continued)

e How are you taking care of the problem(s) now? _____
_____

f What makes the problem(s) better? _____
_____

g What makes the problem(s) worse? _____
_____

h What are your goals for physical therapy?_____
_____

i Are you seeing anyone else for the problem(s)? (Check all that apply)

(1) ☐ Acupuncturist
(2) ☐ Cardiologist
(3) ☐ Chiropractor
(4) ☐ Dentist
(5) ☐ Family practitioner
(6) ☐ Internist
(7) ☐ Massage therapist
(8) ☐ Neurologist
(9) ☐ Obstetrician/gynecologist

(10) ☐ Occupational therapist
(11) ☐ Orthopedist
(12) ☐ Osteopath
(13) ☐ Pediatrician
(14) ☐ Podiatrist
(15) ☐ Primary care physician
(16) ☐ Rheumatologist
Other:_____

24 FUNCTIONAL STATUS/ACTIVITY LEVEL (Check all that apply):

a ☐ Difficulty with locomotion/movement:
(1) ☐ bed mobility
(2) ☐ transfers (such as moving from bed to chair, from bed to commode)
(3) ☐ gait (walking)
(a) ☐ on level (c) ☐ on ramps
(b) ☐ on stairs (d) ☐ on uneven terrain
b ☐ Difficulty with self-care (such as bathing, dressing, eating, toileting)
c ☐ Difficulty with home management (such as household chores, shopping, driving/transportation, care of dependents)
d ☐ Difficulty with community and work activities/integration
(1) ☐ work/school
(2) ☐ recreation or play activity

25 MEDICATIONS

a Do you take any prescription medications? (1) ☐ Yes (2) ☐ No
If yes, please list: _____

b Do you take any nonprescription medications? (Check all that apply)

(1) ☐ Advil/Aleve
(2) ☐ Antacids
(3) ☐ Ibuprofen/ Naproxen
(4) ☐ Antihistamines
(5) ☐ Aspirin

(6) ☐ Decongestants
(7) ☐ Herbal supplements
(8) ☐ Tylenol
(9) ☐ Other:_____
_____

c Have you taken any medications previously for the condition for which you are seeing the physical therapist?
(1) ☐ Yes (2) ☐ No If yes, please list:_____

26 OTHER CLINICAL TESTS—Within the past year, have you had any of the following tests? (Check all that apply)

a ☐ Angiogram
b ☐ Arthroscopy
c ☐ Biopsy
d ☐ Blood tests
e ☐ Bone scan
f ☐ Bronchoscopy
g ☐ CT scan
h ☐ Doppler ultrasound
i ☐ Echocardiogram
j ☐ EEG (electroencephalogram)
k ☐ EKG (electrocardiogram)
l ☐ EMG (electromyogram)

m ☐ Mammogram
n ☐ MRI
o ☐ Myelogram
p ☐ NCV (nerve conduction velocity)
q ☐ Pap smear
r ☐ Pulmonary function test
s ☐ Spinal tap
t ☐ Stool tests
u ☐ Stress test (e.g., treadmill, bicycle)
v ☐ Urine tests
x ☐ X-rays
y ☐ Other:_____

© American Physical Therapy Association 1999; revised September 2000, January 2002

DOCUMENTATION TEMPLATE FOR
PHYSICAL THERAPIST PATIENT/CLIENT MANAGEMENT
Systems Review

	Not Impaired	Impaired
CARDIOVASCULAR/PULMONARY SYSTEM	☐	☐

Heart rate: _____

Respiratory rate: _____

Blood pressure: _____

Edema: _____

	Not Impaired	Impaired
INTEGUMENTARY SYSTEM	☐	☐

Integrity
    Pliability (texture): _____
    Presence of scar formation: _____
    Skin color: _____
    Skin integrity: _____

	Not Impaired	Impaired
MUSCULOSKELETAL SYSTEM		
Gross Symmetry	☐	☐

    Standing: _____
    Sitting: _____
    Activity specific: _____

	Not Impaired	Impaired
Gross Range of Motion	☐	☐
Gross Strength	☐	☐

Other: _____

```
┌─────────────────────────────────┐
│  Height  _____   │
│                                  │
│  Weight  _____   │
└─────────────────────────────────┘
```

NEUROMUSCULAR SYSTEM
Gross Coordinated Movements

	Not Impaired	Impaired
Balance	☐	☐
Gait	☐	☐
Locomotion	☐	☐
Transfers	☐	☐
Transitions	☐	☐
Motor function (motor control, motor learning)	☐	☐

COMMUNICATION, AFFECT, COGNITION, LEARNING STYLE

	Not Impaired	Impaired
Communication (e.g., age-appropriate)	☐	☐
Orientation x 3 (person/place/time)	☐	☐
Emotional/behavioral responses	☐	☐

Learning barriers:
☐ None
☐ Vision
☐ Hearing
☐ Unable to read
☐ Unable to understand what is read
☐ Language/needs interpreter
☐ Other: _____

Education needs:
☐ Disease process
☐ Safety
☐ Use of devices/equipment
☐ Activities of daily living
☐ Exercise program
☐ Other: _____

How does patient/client best learn? ☐ Pictures ☐ Reading ☐ Listening ☐ Demonstration ☐ Other: _____

DOCUMENTATION TEMPLATE FOR
PHYSICAL THERAPIST PATIENT/CLIENT MANAGEMENT
Tests and Measures

KEY TO TESTS AND MEASURES:

1 Aerobic Capacity/Endurance
2 Anthropometric Characteristics
3 Arousal, Attention, and Cognition
4 Assistive and Adaptive Devices
5 Circulation (Arterial, Venous, Lymphatic)
6 Cranial and Peripheral Nerve Integrity
7 Environmental, Home, and Work (Job/School/Play) Barriers
8 Ergonomics and Body Mechanics
9 Gait, Locomotion, and Balance
10 Integumentary Integrity
11 Joint Integrity and Mobility
12 Motor Function (Motor Control and Motor Learning)
13 Muscle Performance (Including Strength, Power, and Endurance)

14 Neuromotor Development and Sensory Integration
15 Orthotic, Protective, and Supportive Devices
16 Pain
17 Posture
18 Prosthetic Requirements
19 Range of Motion (Including Muscle Length)
20 Reflex Integrity
21 Self-Care and Home Management (Including Activities of Daily Living and Instrumental Activities of Daily Living)
22 Sensory Integrity
23 Ventilation and Respiration/Gas Exchange
24 Work (Job/School/Play), Community, and Leisure Integration or Reintegration (Including Instrumental Activities of Daily Living)

NOTES:

DOCUMENTATION TEMPLATE FOR
PHYSICAL THERAPIST PATIENT/CLIENT MANAGEMENT
Evaluation

DIAGNOSIS:

Musculoskeletal Patterns

☐ A: Primary Prevention/Risk Reduction for Skeletal Demineralization

☐ B: Impaired Posture

☐ C: Impaired Muscle Performance

☐ D: Impaired Joint Mobility, Motor Function, Muscle Performance, and Range of Motion Associated With Connective Tissue Dysfunction

☐ E: Impaired Joint Mobility, Motor Function, Muscle Performance, and Range of Motion Associated With Localized Inflammation

☐ F: Impaired Joint Mobility, Motor Function, Muscle Performance, Range of Motion, and Reflex Integrity Associated With Spinal Disorders

☐ G: Impaired Joint Mobility, Muscle Performance, and Range of Motion Associated With Fracture

☐ H: Impaired Joint Mobility, Motor Function, Muscle Performance, and Range of Motion Associated With Joint Arthroplasty

☐ I: Impaired Joint Mobility, Motor Function, Muscle Performance, and Range of Motion Associated With Bony or Soft Tissue Surgery

☐ J: Impaired Motor Function, Muscle Performance, Range of Motion, Gait, Locomotion, and Balance Associated With Amputation

Neuromuscular Patterns

☐ A: Primary Prevention/Risk Reduction for Loss of Balance and Falling

☐ B: Impaired Neuromotor Development

☐ C: Impaired Motor Function and Sensory Integrity Associated With Nonprogressive Disorders of the Central Nervous System— Congenital Origin or Acquired in Infancy or Childhood

☐ D: Impaired Motor Function and Sensory Integrity Associated With Nonprogressive Disorders of the Central Nervous System— Acquired in Adolescence or Adulthood

☐ E: Impaired Motor Function and Sensory Integrity Associated With Progressive Disorders of the Central Nervous System

☐ F: Impaired Peripheral Nerve Integrity and Muscle Performance Associated With Peripheral Nerve Injury

☐ G: Impaired Motor Function and Sensory Integrity Associated With Acute or Chronic Polyneuropathies

☐ H: Impaired Motor Function, Peripheral Nerve Integrity, and Sensory Integrity Associated With Nonprogressive Disorders of the Spinal Cord

☐ I: Impaired Arousal, Range of Motion, and Motor Control Associated With Coma, Near Coma, or Vegetative State

Cardiovascular/Pulmonary Patterns

☐ A: Primary Prevention/Risk Reduction for Cardiovascular/Pulmonary Disorders

☐ B: Impaired Aerobic Capacity/Endurance Associated With Deconditioning

☐ C: Impaired Ventilation, Respiration/Gas Exchange, and Aerobic Capacity/Endurance Associated With Airway Clearance Dysfunction

☐ D: Impaired Aerobic Capacity/Endurance Associated With Cardiovascular Pump Dysfunction or Failure

☐ E: Impaired Ventilation and Respiration/Gas Exchange Associated With Ventilatory Pump Dysfunction or Failure

☐ F: Impaired Ventilation and Respiration/Gas Exchange Associated With Respiratory Failure

☐ G: Impaired Ventilation, Respiration/Gas Exchange, and Aerobic Capacity/Endurance Associated With Respiratory Failure in the Neonate

☐ H: Impaired Circulation and Anthropometric Dimensions Associated With Lymphatic System Disorders

Integumentary Patterns

☐ A: Primary Prevention/Risk Reduction for Integumentary Disorders

☐ B: Impaired Integumentary Integrity Associated With Superficial Skin Involvement

☐ C: Impaired Integumentary Integrity Associated With Partial-Thickness Skin Involvement and Scar Formation

☐ D: Impaired Integumentary Integrity Associated With Full-Thickness Skin Involvement and Scar Formation

☐ E: Impaired Integumentary Integrity Associated With Skin Involvement Extending Into Fascia, Muscle, or Bone and Scar Formation

PROGNOSIS: _____

_____

_____

_____

_____

_____

_____

_____

_____

_____

_____

DOCUMENTATION TEMPLATE FOR
PHYSICAL THERAPIST PATIENT/CLIENT MANAGEMENT
Plan of Care

Plan of Care

American Physical Therapy Association

Anticipated Goals: _____

_____

_____

_____

Expected Outcomes: _____

_____

_____

_____

Interventions: _____

_____

_____

_____

**Frequency of Visits/Duration
of Episode of Care:**

_____

_____

_____

Education (including safety, exercise, and disease information): _____

_____

_____

Who was educated? ☐ Patient/client ☐ Family (name and relationship): _____
How did patient/family demonstrate learning:
  ☐ Patient/client verbalizes understanding
  ☐ Family/significant other verbalizes understanding
  ☐ Patient/client demonstrates correctly
  ☐ Demonstration is unsuccessful (describe): _____

_____

_____

Discharge Plan: _____

_____

_____

_____

_____

_____

_____

_____

F

Goal Writing Exercise

Rewrite the following general goals into objective, measurable goals.

1. Decrease congestion

2. Improve standing posture

3. Independent with home exercises

4. Increase shoulder movements, all planes by 10 degrees

5. Decrease low back pain

6. Improve ambulation skills

7. Improve cervical rotation

8. Maximize functional ability

9. Decrease UE flexion synergy

10. Patient will be able to sit up

11. Improve motor planning

12. Reduce edema of the LUE

13. Increase endurance

14. Maintain spinal segment in place

15. Control balance

G

Note Writing Exercise

1. Rewrite the following SOAP note in acceptable content format as a SOAP note.
2. Rewrite the following SOAP note in a narrative format with appropriate content and categorize the information.

NOTE # 1:
S: Fixed the lawnmower this weekend
O: Seen in dept. for cont with cybex protocol to BLE's 2 cycles r, 1 cycle L. Followed by balance beam, kicking ball, unilateral stance 15 sec. L unable to maintain L. Side <> side stepping. Side <> side gallop. Fast walking length of speech hall and back 196 in 45 sec 1st trial, 43 in 2nd, 36 in 3rd with encouragement. Kneeling–1/2 kneeling on mat 2 sets 10 reps. Amb 60' with 8 hyperextensions 1st time, 4 2nd, 8 3rd.
A: Tol Rx well, fatigued with ex.
P: Continue

Note # 2:

S: Good spirits

O: Gait + advanced gait + balance techniques – instruction + practice.

A: Demonstrating good gait and balance with some proprioceptive L/E deficit + thus would advise to contact guard stand-by assistance for safety at present.

P: Continue as above

1. Write a chart entry for a patient that did not come to therapy today and did not call to cancel.

2. A patient is brought to PT but refuses to do anything and is disrupting others.

Documentation Content Exercise

For the following intervention entries, please answer the following:

1. Is it written objectively with all appropriate objective information included?
2. Is the terminology correct for reimbursement and billing?
3. Is the intervention reproducible based on the information given?
4. If there is enough information to reproduce the treatment, defend your decision.
5. If there is not enough information to reproduce the treatment, what other information do you need?

1. Strengthening exercises to the LEs.

2. Massage to neck

3. Electrical stimulation to low back

4. Joint mobilization lumbar region

5. Gait training

6. Intermittent cervical traction in supine, head in neutral × 20 minutes, 25 pounds, 30 second hold, 15 second release

7. Stretching to R heelcords

8. Biofeedback for R UE

9. US to L calf

10. Back exercises

I

Physical Therapy
Note Examples

Appendix I

Physical Therapy Evaluation

Name: Grant Stern   **Date:** 10/26/04
DOB: 2/19/68   **SS#:** 213-36-8245
Referring Physician: M. Sandhouse, D.O.
Diagnosis: Medical: 820.9 fracture of neck of femur, unspecified, open L
PT treatment diagnosis: 781.2 gait abnormality (orthopedic)

Medical History: See attached General History for additional information.
34 y.o. male referred 10/25/04 with L femur fracture, s/p ORIF, hip pinning, 10/5/04 secondary to auto accident 10/04/04. Patient was a passenger. Hospitalized at BGMC 10/4 to 10/22/04. Other injuries included: multiple abrasions and lacerations extremities and face, which are in various stages of healing. No other medical problems prior to accident.
Meds: Percocet, PRN, Tylenol PRN for pain.
Social history: Married, lives in 2 story townhouse with stairs, bedrooms on second floor. 2 children, ages 3 and 5. Vocation: Middle school teacher in Broward County, but currently not working. Drives car with automatic transmission. Leisure: mountain biking, running.
Chief complaints: Unable to sleep, dependent on walker, unable to work, unable to enjoy leisure activities, unable to play with kids.
Precautions: 50% WB LLE
Barriers to learning: none
Home Barriers: stairs
Cognition:
    Intact, appropriate communication, accurate historian
Vital signs at rest: BP: 130 / 80   P: 84   RR: 16
Vitals following eval session: BP: 132 / 84   P: 86   RR: 18
Endurance:
    Becomes SOB with exertion. Requires 1 minute of rest for every 5 minutes of activity.
Pain:
    L hip: at rest 5/10, wakes him up at night 3 to 4x, when changes position
    With WB: 9/10   With movement: 8/10
Integument/Sensation:
    Surgical incision L lateral hip, staples out, incision closed, dark pink in appearance. Lacks sensation to light touch/pain along incision. Intact otherwise. Scabs on face and both lower extremities. No open areas noted.
    Mild edema in area of incision.
    Proprioception intact UEs & LEs.
DTRs:
    Normal

ADL: Per patient, I in toileting (elevated toilet seat) and showering. Uses shower chair at home with hand held shower head. I in self-feeding. Dresses in sitting using reacher and sock aid.

Mobility: Drove self to therapy, has compact type car.

Bed mobility: I rolling L/R, scooting up and down, scooting L/R.

Transfers: I: sit to supine, sit to stand, stand pivot using front wheel rolling walker (FWRW) and without, PWB 50% LLE. Able to transfer toward R and toward L, also I in all car transfers.

Gait: I with FWRW, 50% WB LLE on even surfaces and carpet. Demonstrates minimal WB on LLE with short stance, decreased stride and step length and step to pattern. Speed slow, at 40 meters per minute. Flexed posture with walker. Tendency to turn toward R, avoiding directional changes to L when possible. Initial contact with foot flat. Decreased hip flexion in swing phase. Distance limited to 50 to 75' (household).

Unable to negotiate stairs in upright, and has been going up and down at home in sitting, bumping up and down on buttocks once per day.

Balance:

Stable with FWRW

Without walker: Single leg stance on R x 2 seconds with balance loss to left, able to I recover.

Strength:

UE s:	gross strength	5/5
RLE:	gross strength	5/5
LLE:	Hip flexion	2/5
	Abduction	2-/5
	Knee flexion	3-/5
	Extension	3-/5
	Ankle dorsiflexion	5/5
	Plantarflexion	~4-/5

Range of Motion:

UE s: no deficits noted, intact

RLE: no deficits noted, intact

		Active	Passive
LLE:	hip flexion	100°	120° with pain
	Abduction	10°	15°
	Adduction	to neutral	to neutral
	External rotation	10°	10°
	Internal rotation	10°	10°
	Knee flexion	80°	100°
	Extension	-5°	0°

| Ankle dorsiflexion | 8° | 15° |
| Plantarflexion | 40° | 40° |

Problem Summary:
Weakness LLE, ROM deficits LLE, Balance deficit in standing, Pain LLE, Gait walker dependent on even surfaces only, Abnormal gait pattern, Flexed posture in standing, endurance limitations, limited weight bearing

Gait limited to indoor surfaces primarily, household ambulator, unable to negotiate stairs in upright, unable to balance in upright for upright activities such as shaving, dresses in sit with assistive devices, fatigue secondary to inability to sleep through night, requires frequent rest during activity

Unable to work, unable to participate in play with children, unable to socialize or engage in leisure activities

Goals:
STGs: 11/08/04
Patient will be able to achieve gait with FWRW 200 feet on even and carpeted surfaces for safe standing in self-care.
Single leg stance on R x 20 seconds with balance loss to left, able to I recover.
MMT LLE: Hip flexion   3/5, Abduction   3/5

LTGs: 12/6/04
Patient will be able to achieve gait 200 feet with a straight cane on even surfaces, carpeted surfaces, and outdoors.
MMT LLE: Hip flexion   4/5, Abduction   4-/5
L Knee flexion   AROM 100°   PROM 130°
Return to work with straight cane
Requires 1 minute of rest for every 25 minutes of activity.

P: OP PT x 3 /week for 4 weeks to consist of gait training with FWRW and cane, crutches, progressive ther ex, neuromuscular re-ed, and cold pack LLE.

Signature: *Regina Brown*, PT 00723

SOAP Daily Note – Out-patient

Pt Name: Grant Stern   Date: 11/06/04
Time: 1:00 pm to 2:15 pm

Diagnosis: Medical: 820.9 fracture of neck of femur, unspecified, open L
PT treatment diagnosis: 781.2 gait abnormality (orthopedic)
Guide Section: 4H, 4I

S: Pt stated "Able to sleep through the night up to 6 hours now, as pain in my hip is no longer waking me up."
O: Precautions: PWB 50% LLE
24 minutes: 97116: Gait training: x3 trials each, contact guard with axillary crutches 4 point pattern; even surface x50 feet, grass, carpet, training stairs, 5 up/down; ascended/descended using crutches contact guard with verbal cues for crutch placement, and pattern. Tendency to for initial contact on left with whole foot, short stance on left without verbal cues.
15 minutes: 97110: Therapeutic exercise: in standing: Active: L hip abduction, adduction, flexion, extension, circumduction x10 reps each, rest in between, holding handrail. Supine: Active L knee extension hamstring stretch x2, 30 sec hold, quad sets/glut sets bilaterally: x5 reps, 20 sec hold. Strength: L hip flexion 3+/5; abduction 3+/5.
18 minutes: 97112: Neuromuscular re-education: Balance training without crutches: single leg stance on R, eyes open minimal assist 10% (or limited assist 10%) for balance. Balance loss to the left, after 10 secs, 10 reps. Assist required to right self.
15 minutes: 97010: Cold pack L hip patient in R sidelying, pillow between knees for comfort following gait and exercise. Instructed to use axillary crutches at home instead of FWRW, on indoor surfaces only at present for safety and to continue with home exercises as previously instructed.

A: Progressed from front wheeled rolling walker to axillary crutches in order to increase mobility on uneven surfaces, including curbs and stairs. Skin on hip intact prior and following application of cold pack, mild hyperemia present. Patient is progressing toward his established goals of I on all surfaces with crutches, as well as increasing the strength of the L hip musculature.

P: Will continue with OP PT x 3/week for gait training, progressive ther ex, neuromuscular re-ed and cold pack. Plan to add resistance for ther ex next visit, 2#s.

Signature: *Lynn Robert*, PT 0001234

For billing purposes: Non-Medicare

Diagnosis: Medical: 820.9 fracture of neck of femur, unspecified, open L

PT treatment diagnosis: 781.2 gait abnormality (orthopedic)

Codes:	Procedures:	Units:
97116	Gait training	1 unit (based on a 15 minute unit)
97110	Therapeutic ex	1 unit (based on a 15 minute unit)
97112	Neuromuscular re-ed	1 unit (based on a 15 minute unit)
97010	Cold pack	1 unit (based on a 15 minute unit)

AUTHOR'S NOTE

Non-Medicare. *Although gait training was 24 minutes, as AMA CPT codes/procedures are in 15-minute increments, it only qualifies as one unit. The session qualifies for 4 units of care.*

Medicare. *Under Medicare coding guidelines, cold packs cannot be charged as individual procedures. Although they must be included in the documentation, they are not separately reimbursable as they are considered "bundled." Additionally, from a time perspective, as Medicare unit ranges from 8 to 23 minutes, each procedure qualifies for 1 unit, for a total of 3 units. For billing of services in SNFs, the terms limited assist and extensive assist are recommended by CMS with %s, for what were previously minimal assist and maximal assist. Regardless of the terminology used, however, the % of assist needed or % of patient/client dependence, must be included as well as a description of the behavior or dysfunction that characterizes the assistance needed.*

Narrative Daily Note – Out-patient

Grant Stern
Drives I to visits, ambulatory with FWRW.

11/06/04
1:00 – 2:15 pm: Patient s/p L femur fracture, I ambulator with FWRW PWB to PT for
97116 Gait training: 3 trials each, contact guard with axillary crutches 4 point pattern,
PWB LLE 50% on even surface x 50 feet, grass, carpet, training stairs; 5 up and down.
Contact guard and verbal cues for correct pattern and crutch placement. Short stance on
L, initial contact L with whole foot.
97110 Therapeutic exercise: in standing, active, for L hip abduction, L hip adduction,
flexion, extension, circumduction x 10 reps each, rest in between, holding handrail.
Supine: Active L knee extension hamstring stretch x2, 30 sec hold, quad sets/glut sets
bilaterally: x5 reps, 20 sec hold. Strength: L hip flexion 3+/5; abduction 3+/5.
97112 Neuromuscular re-education: Balance training without crutches: single leg stance
on R, eyes open minimal assist 10% (or limited assist 10%) for balance. Balance loss to
the left, after 10 secs, 10 reps. Assist required to right self.
97010 Cold pack L hip x 15 minutes, patient in R sidelying, pillow between knees for
comfort following gait and exercise. Reported pain level at 6/10 prior to CP and 3/10
following. Skin intact before and after with mild hyperemia after.
Pt. stated that he's able to sleep up to 6 hours per night now.
Instructed to use axillary crutches at home, instead of FWRW, on indoor surfaces only at
present for safety and to continue with home exercises as previously instructed.
Demonstrating steady improvement as evidenced by progression from FWRW to
crutches. Will continue with OP PT x 3/week for gait training, progressive ther ex,
neuromuscular re-ed and cold pack. Plan to add resistance for ther ex next visit, 2#s.

Signature: *Lynn Robert*, PT

0001234

Flowsheet Example 1

Pt: Grant Stern

Please indicate # of units as applicable for each procedure (or a check ✓ if units are non-billable) and initials of individual treating

Procedure	11/06/04										
Gait training 97116	1 ℒℛ										
Ther ex 97110	1 ℒℛ										
Neuro-muscular re-ed 97112	1 ℒℛ										
Cold pack 97010	1 ℒℛ										
Home Instruction	✓ ℒℛ										
Supplemental entries by date:											

11/06/04:

Progressed from FWRW to axillary crutches: CG & VC: ascend and descend 5 steps, grass, carpet, even surface 50', x 3 reps each. Ther ex, active in standing L hip: in all planes, 10 reps, single leg stance R, 10 secs with balance loss to L. CP L hip in sidelying at end of session x 15 mins. Pain ▼ from 6/10 to 3/10 following CP. Add 2# resistance next visit, cont 3x/week. *Lynn Robert*, PT 0001234

Flowsheet Example 2

Pt: Grant Stern

Please indicate # of units as applicable for each procedure (or a check ✓ if units are non-billable) and initials of individual treating

Procedure	11/06/04									
Gait training 97116 **FWRW** **crutches** **even** **carpet** **stairs** **curbs** **grass**	1 *PP* ✓ ✓ ✓ ✓ ✓									
Ther ex 97110 **Active** **Standing** **Supine** **Sidelying** **Prone** **Resistive** **Standing** **Supine** **Sidelying** **Prone**	1 *LR* ✓ ✓									
Neuro-muscular re-ed 97112 **Balance**	1 *LR* ✓									
Cold pack 97010	1 *LR*									
Home Instruction	✓ *LR*									

Supplemental entries by date:

11/06/04:
Progressed from FWRW to axillary crutches: CG & VC: ascend and descend 5 steps, grass, carpet, even surface 50', x 3 reps each. Ther ex, active in standing L hip: in all planes, 10 reps, single leg stance R, 10 secs with balance loss to L. CP L hip in sidelying at end of session x 15 mins. Pain ▼ from 6/10 to 3/10 following CP. Add 2# resistance next visit, cont 3x/week. *Lynn Robert*, PT 0001234

Clinical Pathway Example

Medical Diagnosis:

820.9 fracture of neck of femur, unspecified, open L

PT Diagnosis:

781.2 gait abnormality (orthopedic)

Weight bearing status: FWB RLE   **PWB 50%** LLE

PT: Name: Print Jennifer Allan   **Signature:** *Jennifer Allan*   **Initials:**

JA, DPT

PT: Name: Print: Lynn Robert   **Signature:** *Lynn Robert*   **Initials:** *LR*

PT

PT: Name: Print: _____ **Signature**_____**Initials:** _____

	Gait training 97116	Gait training	Gait training	Gait training	Ther ex 97110	Ther ex	Ther ex	Instructions
Date	I crutches even surface	I crutches carpet	I crutches grass/ outdoor	I crutches stairs	3/5 strength L hip: ✓, abd	3+/5 strength L hip: ✓, abd	4-/5 strength L hip: ✓, abd	I HEP
11/02/04					✓ *JA*			✓ *JA*
11/06/04	✓ *LR*					✓ *LR*		✓ *LR*

Discharge status:

Interim supplemental entries as indicated:

11/02/04:

Progressed from FWRW to axillary crutches 4 point gait: CG & VC: even surface 50', x 3 reps. Ther ex, active on mat in antigravity positions: L hip: in all planes, 10 reps, single leg stance R, 5 secs with balance loss to L. Able to sleep 4 hours uninterrupted by pain. Progress to ther ex in standing next visit, cont 3x/week. *Jennifer Allan,* **DPT 0002234**

11/06/04:

Progressed from FWRW to axillary crutches: CG & VC: ascend and descend 5 steps, grass, carpet, even surface 50', x 3 reps each. Ther ex, active in standing L hip: in all planes, 10 reps, single leg stance R, 10 secs with balance loss to L. CP L hip in sidelying at end of session x 15 mins. Pain ▾ from 6/10 to 3/10 following CP. Able to sleep up to 6 hours now. Add 2# resistance next visit, cont 3x/week. *Lynn Robert,* **PT 0001234**

Index

Page numbers followed by the letters *f* and *t* indicate figures and tables, respectively.

ADL (activities of daily living), documenting, 119–120
ADL index score, MDS and, 93, 95*t*
American Health Information Management Association (AHIMA), health record and, 3
Anthropometric, 110
APTA (American Physical Therapy Association)
  coding and, 44
  continuation of care and, 39–41
  Guide for Professional Conduct v. models for, 89–90
  Guide to Physical Therapist Practice and, 24
  progress notes and, 40
APTA guidelines, Medicare documentation v., 27
Ashworth Scale, utilization support with, 161
Assessment reference dates (ARD), MDS and, 95
Authentication
  law and, 82
  Medicare inclusions in, 36–37
Authorization, claim denials and, 18

Billing, 5
  EMR and, 147–148
Body mechanics, evaluation of, 119
Borg's perceived exertion scale, measurements and, 160
Bundling, codes and, 46–47

Centers for Medicare and Medicaid (CMS). *See also* Medicare; Medicaid; CMS Medicare Carrier Manual
  documentation and, 2
Claims, insurance
  hearings for, 167
  non-covered conditions and, 18
Clinical Decision-Making model (CDMM), 24, 26*t*, 28
Clinical tools, physical therapy and, 23
CMS. *See* Centers for Medicare and Medicaid (CMS)
CMS Medicare Carrier Manual, guidelines in, 59–60, 63–70
Codes. *See also* CPT (current procedural terminology; HCPCS) codes; ICD-9-diagnosis order
  bundling of, 46, 47
  individual, 44–45
  modifiers and, 46
  principles of using, 44
  procedure specificity and, 45–46
  therapeutic procedures and, 47–55
  time and, 46
Cognition, diagnostic testing and, 158
Computer-based patient record (CPR), 3
Confidentiality, 74–76
Continuation of care
  documentation of, 39–41
  intervention plan in, 110, 110*t*
  pediatrics and, 130–131

Countersignature, 81–82
CPT (current procedural terminology; HCPCS) codes, 13, 44
  matching codes and, 45
  overview of, 43
Critical (clinical) pathways, therapy plan and, 24, 25*t*

Data, Evaluation, Performance Goals (DEP) format, 22, 23
Data types, 12
Demographic information, documentation of, 157
Denials (claims), reasons for, 17–18
Device use. *See also* Orthotics; Prosthesis
  documentation of, 36
Diagnosis, 34
  PT and, 28–29
  relevance of, 156
Diagnostic testing, documentation in, 158
Direct data entry (DDE) system, overview of, 166
Disablement models, categories in, 27*t*, 28
Discharge summary, 174*t*–175*t*
  APTA summation and, 40
Disclosure, improper, legal issues and, 85
Documentation
  APTA and, 34*t*
  continuation of care and, 161–162
  episode of care and, 162–163
  initial examination and, 33–34
  Medicare and, 34*t*
  patient care and, 71
  patient restraint use and, 89
  reexamination and, 162–163
  requirements for, 33
  special concerns in, 84–85
  UR practices and, 154–155
Documentation by exception, record keeping and, 24

Edema, documentation of, 118
Electronic claims, 86
Electronic mail, risk management and, 86
Electronic medical record (EMR), 3
  documentation with, 143–144
  overview of, 139–140, 150–151
  system architecture of, 140–142
    clinical reports and, 145*f*
    clinician list and, 150*f*
    laptop computer in, 141*f*
    objective documentation screen in, 142*f*
  training and support in using, 142–143
Endurance scale, 120*t*
Essential functional activities (EFA), 36

Evaluation (patient)
    documentation and, 33–34
    PT and, 29
Examination, patient
    documentation and, 156–157, 170t–172t
    PT and, 29
External review, overview of, 164–168

Flowsheets, 23, 24t
Focus on Therapeutic Outcomes, Inc. (FOTO), 23, 40
Formats, individual entry. *See* Individual entry formats
Functional diagnosis, Medicare and, 18
Functional independence measure (FIM), 23, 40
Functional Outcome Report (FOR) format, 22, 23

Gross motor development, pediatric patient and, 128
Guide to Physical Therapist Practice
    APTA models and, 24
    categories of tests in, 103
    goals and expected outcomes in, 106, 107t, 108t, 109

Health Insurance Portability and Accountability Act, medical
        record and, 5
Health records. *See also* Documentation; Legal Proceedings
    accuracy in, 13
    authentication of, 14
    content inclusion within, 15
    courtesy within, 14–15
    denial issues and, 17–18
    destruction of, 82–83
    documentation problems in, 77–79
    errors in, 12
    formats for, 21–22
    functions and users of, 3, 5, 6t, 7t, 8
    general principles for, 11
    grammar in, 13
    individual charts and, 11–12
    as legal document, 72, 76–77, 86–88
    legibility of, 12
    purposes of, 1–3, 4t, 5t
    referral information and, 11
    storage of, 11
    summary of, 8–9
    timeliness of entry in, 12–13

ICD-9 diagnosis order, 13, 44–45
    matching codes and, 45
Identification information, 34
Incidence reports, 81
Individual entry formats, variety of, 22–23
Informed consent
    overview of, 80–81
    plan of care and, 156
Initial visit, documentation for, 34–36
Institute of Medicine, users of health records and, 8
Insurance. *See also* Claims, insurance; Medicare; Medicaid;
        Third party payer
    pediatrics and, 134t, 135–136
Interventions
    documentation of, 121–122
    identification of, 162
    PT and, 30

Joint Commission on Accreditation of Healthcare
        Organizations (JCAHO), 8
Joint integrity and mobility. *See also* Range of Motion (ROM)
    components of, 117–119
    examples of, 111–117

Law, statutes and, 73
Legal proceedings, professional liability and, 88

Malpractice, medical
    documentation and, 72
    overview of, 72
Managed care, documentation and, 2
MDS. *See* Minimum data set (MDS)
Medicaid, pediatrics and, 133, 134t
Medical history, 34
Medical practice, records and, 1
Medical records. *See* Health records
Medicare
    appeal process in, 166–168
    APTA guidelines v., 2
    components of, 166-168
    documentation and, 2
    inpatient v. outpatient billing with, 104–106
    non-covered services and, 18
    pediatrics and, 134t
    PT services and, 61–63
    reasonable and necessary care with, 165
    recertification documentation and, 39
    state to state eligibility for, 60–61
    tests and measures in, 103
    UR and, 154
Medications, documentation of, 157
Minimum data set (MDS)
    personnel reporting on, 91
    prospective payment system and, 91–92
    special treatments in, 96–99
Modalities, codes and, 46
Modifiers, codes and, 46

Nagi disablement model, documentation in, 155
Noncompliance, 81

Objective data, POMR and, 21
Occupational therapy, co-treatment and, 65
Orthotics
    documentation for, 117
    types of, 120
Outcomes assessment, PT and, 30

Pain chart, medical records and, 16f
Pain reduction, functional performance and, 122
Patient care
    abandonment of, 73–74
    management of, 5
    PT and, 29
    support and, 5
Patient care providers, 8
Pediatrics
    assessment of, 129–130
    initial examination in, 123–129
        history during, 124t–126t

Peer review organizations (PROs), evolution of, 154
Physical restraints, documentation of, 89
Physical therapists (PTs), documentation and, 3
Physical therapy (outpatient), plan of care and, 37–38
Physical therapy (PT)
   diagnosis in, 34
   history of record keeping and, 2
   types of services covered in, 63
Physician's certification, content of, 38
Plan of care (POC), 36–37
   pediatrics and, 130
Problem, Status, and Plan (PSP) format, 22
Problem, Status, Plan, and Functional Goals (PSPG)
     format, 22
Problem-oriented medical record system (POMR), overview
     of, 21
Professional negligence, 73
Prognosis, PT and, 30
Progress notes, 172t
Prosthesis, types of, 120
Provider eligibility requirements, pediatrics and, 132t

Range of motion (ROM)
   muscle performance and, 161
   neuromuscular measurement and, 161
   pediatric assessment for, 127–128
Recertification documentation, coverage and limitations for,
     38–39
Records. *See* Health Records
Reexamination, 173t
Referral information, 34
Rehabilitation services, skilled, 67–70
Reimbursement, 5
   authorized providers and, 150
   coding and, 43
   documentation and, 89
   pediatric PT and, 131–133
Relative value resource based systems (RVRBS), overview
     of, 43
Release of health information, 76
Reporting schedule, 99t
Research
   disclosure of medical information for, 83–84
   treatment duration and, 149
Resident assessment protocol (RAP), 98t
   quality indicators within, 97, 98t
Resource utilization groups (RUGS)
   categories of, 92–93, 92t
   time and frequency requirements for, 94t
Review worksheet, therapy content, 169

Reviewer, third party payer, therapy content worksheet for, 168t
Risk management, 85–86
   videotaped patient care records and, 88
RPTs (return to providers), reasons for, 166
RUGS. *See* Resource utilization groups (RUGS)

Secondary diagnosis, significance of, 157
Signed consent, 34
Skilled services, teaching and training activities and, 67–70
Skin integrity, utilization and, 160
SOAP progress note, plan and, 21, 22
SOAPIER progress note, plan and, 21, 22
Social history, 35
Source-oriented record keeping system (SOMR), overview
     of, 21
Speech pathology services, plan of care and, 37–38
Standardized forms
   initial examination and, 59
   overview of, 57–58
   terminology in, 58–59
Start of care (SOC) date, 34
Subjective data, POMR and, 21
Summation of care, pediatrics and, 131

Telemedical records, 86
Termination of care, categories of, 163
Terminology, medical
   documentation and, 159, 159t
   PT terms and functional phrase alternatives in, 160t
Tests and measures
   baseline data from, 35–36
   Medicare v. non-Medicare, 103–104
Therapy goals, 35
Third-party payer, claims and, 18
Third party providers, pediatrics and, 134t
Treatment
   documentation of, 121–122
   history of prior, 157–158
   patient goals and, 158

Utilization management (UM), overview of, 153–154, 163–164
Utilization review, 176
   documentation and, 155–156
   reimbursement process and, 157
   summary of tasks in, 168–169
Utilization review organizations (UROs), claims and, 165
Utilization Review Quality Assurance (URQA), 153

Verbal orders, health records and, 15–16

Wounds, documentation and, 118